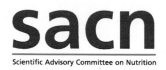

The influence of maternal, fetal and child nutrition on the development of chronic disease in later life

Scientific Advisory Committee on Nutrition

2011

London: TSO

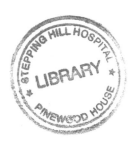

Any enquiries regarding this publication should be sent to the SACN Secretariat: www.sacn.gov.uk/contact_us/index.html

This document is available from the SACN website at www.sacn.gov.uk

ISBN: 9780108510649

Printed in the UK by The Stationery Office Limited

ID P002436882   06/11   10448   19585

Printed on paper containing 75% recycled fibre content minimum.

Preface

The Scientific Advisory Committee on Nutrition's (SACN) Subgroup on Maternal and Child Nutrition (SMCN) has reviewed the evidence that early life nutrition exerts long-term effects and influences the risk of chronic disease in adulthood. It has brought together findings from both observational and experimental studies, considering implications for maternal and child nutrition in the UK. The report was made available for comment in February 2010, and I would like to thank all of those who responded to the consultation.

The Subgroup has concluded that there is cause for concern about the later health consequences of compromised or excessive nutrient supply during early fetal and infant life. It notes that in the context of reproduction, the impact of current dietary patterns on women and girls is of particular concern, and considers that improving the nutritional status of women of childbearing age, infants and young children has the potential to improve the health of future generations. The Committee also offers recommendations for future research in this area, particularly emphasising the need for data which better characterise dietary patterns and patterns of pre and postnatal growth.

I would particularly like to thank Dr Anthony Williams, Chair of the Subgroup, for leading this important piece of work, as well as all members of the Subgroup and Secretariat for their time and valued contribution to this report. I would also like to thank others for their early contribution to this work.

Dr Ann Prentice
Chair of the Scientific Advisory Committee on Nutrition
March 2011

Contents

Membership of Scientific Advisory Committee on Nutrition: Subgroup on Maternal and Child Nutrition (SMCN):

Chair:

Dr Anthony F Williams — Reader in Child Nutrition & Consultant in Neonatal Paediatrics, St George's, University of London

Members:

Professor Peter Aggett — Honorary Professor, School of Medicine and Health Lancaster University

Professor Annie S Anderson — Professor of Food Choice, Centre for Public Health Nutrition Research, University of Dundee

Dr Robert Fraser — Reader, Reproductive and Developmental Medicine University of Sheffield

Professor Alan A Jackson — Professor of Human Nutrition, School of Medicine, University of Southampton

Professor Timothy Key — Professor in Epidemiology and Deputy Director of Cancer Epidemiology Unit, University of Oxford

Dr Ken Ong
(*from November 2009*) — Paediatric Endocrinologist, Addenbrooke's Hospital; and Affiliated Lecturer, Department of Paediatrics, University of Cambridge

Dr Ann Prentice — Director, Medical Research Council Human Nutrition Research, Cambridge

Dr Sian Robinson
(*from November 2009*) — Principal Research Fellow, MRC Epidemiology Resource Centre, University of Southampton

Dr Stella M Walsh — Postgraduate Programme Leader, Leeds Metropolitan University (lay member)

Observers:

Ruth Campbell	The Scottish Government, Health Department
Susan Sky	The Welsh Assembly, Health Promotion Division
Dr Fiona Bissett	Scottish Government, Health Department

Secretariat:

Dr Sheela Reddy (Scientific)

Rachel Marklew (Scientific)

Lisa Miles (Scientific)

Rachel Elsom (Scientific)

Membership of Scientific Advisory Committee on Nutrition (SACN):

Chair:

Dr Ann Prentice
(*from June 2010*)

Director, Medical Research Council Human Nutrition Research, Cambridge

Professor Alan A Jackson
(*until June 2010*)

Professor of Human Nutrition, School of Medicine, University of Southampton

Members:

Professor Peter Aggett

Honorary Professor, School of Medicine and Health, Lancaster University

Professor Annie S Anderson

Professor of Food Choice, Centre for Public Health Nutrition Research, University of Dundee

Late Professor Sheila Bingham
(*until March 2009*)

Formerly Director, Medical Research Council's Dunn Human Nutrition Unit, Cambridge

Mrs Christine Gratus

Honorary Senior Research Fellow, University of Birmingham, School of Primary Care Clinical Sciences. Former advertising and marketing research director (lay member)

Dr Paul Haggarty

Head of the Nutrition and Epigenetics Group, Rowett Institute of Nutrition and Health, University of Aberdeen, and Honorary Clinical Scientist in Grampian NHS Trust

Professor Timothy Key

Professor in Epidemiology and Deputy Director of Cancer Epidemiology Unit, University of Oxford

Professor Peter Kopelman
(*until November 2010*)

Principal, St George's, University of London

Dr Susan A Lanham-New
(*from November 2009*)

Reader in Nutrition, Division of Nutritional Sciences, Faculty of Health and Medical Sciences, University of Surrey

Professor Julie Lovegrove
(*from November 2009*)

Reader in Nutritional Metabolism and Deputy Director of Institute of Cardiovascular and Metabolic Research, University of Reading

Professor Ian Macdonald

Professor of Metabolic Physiology at the University of Nottingham, and Director of Research at the Faculty of Medicine and Health Sciences

Professor Harry McCardle
(from November 2009)

Deputy Director of Science and the Director of Academic Affairs at the Rowett Institute of Nutrition and Health, University of Aberdeen

Dr David Mela

Senior Scientist and Expertise Group Leader, Unilever Food and Health Research Institute, the Netherlands

Professor Hilary Powers

Professor of Nutritional Biochemistry and Head of Human Nutrition Unit, University of Sheffield

Dr Ann Prentice
(until June 2010)

Director, Medical Research Council Human Nutrition Research, Cambridge

Dr Anita Thomas

Consultant Physician in Acute Medicine and Care of the Elderly, Plymouth Hospitals NHS Trust

Professor Angus Walls
(from November 2009)

Professor of Restorative Dentistry and Director of Research, School and Dental Sciences, Newcastle University

Dr Stella M Walsh

Postgraduate Programme Leader, Leeds Metropolitan University (lay member)

Dr Anthony F Williams

Reader in Child Nutrition & Consultant in Neonatal Paediatrics, St George's, University of London

Professor Ian Young
(from November 2009)

Professor of Medicine and Director of Health, Queen's University Belfast and Associate Medical Director (Research and Development), Belfast Health and Social Care Trust

Observers:

Mrs Maureen Howell

The Welsh Assembly, Health Promotion Division

Dr Naresh Chada

Department of Health, Social Services and Public Safety, Northern Ireland

Dr Alison Tedstone

Department of Health, England

Secretariat:

Dr Sheela Reddy (Scientific)

Dr Elaine Stone (Scientific)

Rachel Marklew (Scientific)

Lisa Miles (Scientific)

Vicki Pyne (Scientific)

Michael Griffin (Administrative)

Other acknowledgements:

The Committee thanks Dr Christopher Owen and colleagues from the Division of Population Health Sciences and Education at St George's, University of London for undertaking an initial review of the epidemiology in 2005 and for their subsequent contributions. The Committee also thanks Dr Peter Sanderson for his contribution to the drafting of the report.

The influence of maternal, fetal and child nutrition on the development of chronic disease in later life

Executive Summary

Introduction

1. Cardiovascular disease, type 2 diabetes and cancer, are leading causes of death in the UK and present a major contemporary public health challenge. The causes are complex. Many environmental exposures modify risk but diet and lifestyle play a significant part. This report examines the contribution of nutritional exposures in early life.

2. Fetal life and early childhood are periods of rapid growth and development (see Chapter 3). Imbalanced nutrient supply at this stage may alter body structure and function in a way that increases risk of chronic disease and, in girls, may modify the ability to meet the nutritional and other stresses of reproduction. The nutritional status of the population therefore has implications for the health of both current and future generations.

3. Human observational evidence demonstrates associations between growth in early life and adult chronic disease risk (see Chapter 4). Experimental evidence suggests that at least some of these associations may be causal and offers insight into mechanisms (see Chapter 5).

Terms of Reference

4. The Department of Health asked the Scientific Advisory Committee on Nutrition (SACN) to:

    - Review the influence of maternal, fetal and child nutrition, including growth and development *in utero* and up to the age of 5 years, on the development of chronic disease in later life in the offspring.

    - Identify opportunities for nutritional intervention that could influence the risk of chronic disease in later life in the offspring.

Methodology (Chapter 2)

5. Evidence was reviewed in accordance with the principles described in the SACN working document, *A Framework for the Evaluation of Evidence* [Scientific Advisory Committee on Nutrition, 2002].

6. Where available, systematic reviews and meta-analyses of relevant studies were considered, with subsequently published individual studies or trials considered separately. In the absence of reviews, relevant retrospective or prospective studies and trials were identified. Finally, SACN considered experimental studies in humans and animals in order to explore mechanisms and exposure-response relationships, which would help the interpretation of associations noted in observational studies. Studies published after 1st January 2010 were not considered.

7. The evidence associating early life nutrition with later risk of chronic disease is variable in quality. Most of the human evidence demonstrates associations that are susceptible to confounding by environmental and behavioural factors at different stages of the life course. Chronic disease risk is also influenced by genetic predisposition to disease and modifiable risk factors acting in adolescence and adulthood.

8. Epidemiological studies involve prospective or retrospective collection of data. These are complementary approaches with different strengths and weaknesses. In retrospective studies, disease outcomes are known but measures of maternal and early life exposures may be weak. Generalisation to contemporary circumstances can also be questionable. Prospective studies more accurately characterise early nutrient exposure and growth but it may be necessary to infer risk by measuring intermediate markers of risk of later health outcomes. However, despite these limitations the epidemiology helps to frame research questions and design empirical approaches to examine possible mechanisms and establish causality.

9. Experimental interventions, mainly in animal models, help to ascribe mechanisms that may explain the associations observed. As with prospective observational studies, the length of the human lifespan places limitations on most existing intervention studies in humans, although markers of later risk, particularly if validated in animal models, may be useful.

10. SACN has not considered the impact of reproduction on the mother's later health, nor the impact on the offspring of smoking, alcohol and other environmental exposures during pregnancy. It nevertheless appreciates these and re-emphasises their importance.

11. SACN has focussed attention on cardiovascular disease, diabetes and cancer as the leading causes of mortality, but recognises that early life nutritional exposures may affect many other outcomes.

Background – Growth in fetal life and infancy (Chapter 3)

12. Normal growth and development is characterised by a regulated increase in the dimensions, mass and functional complexity of tissues and organs. These processes can be disturbed by failure to provide a balanced and sufficient supply of energy and nutrients. It is hypothesised that the resulting changes in pace and timing of early growth alter body composition, metabolic and physiological function, thereby influencing later chronic disease risk (Chapter 3).

13. Experimental studies in animals have identified "critical periods" in early development when alteration of nutrient supply may alter structure and function irreversibly. This phenomenon is called "nutritional programming" (section 3.4.2). Early nutrient supply can thus influence both the composition and distribution of tissues deposited during growth and consequently the attainment of functional or metabolic capacity at the whole body and cellular level.

14. Although widely used as a descriptor of fetal outcome, birthweight is influenced by many variables other than fetal nutrient supply (section 3.2). These include maternal height, weight, parity, ethnicity and exposure to toxins such as alcohol and tobacco smoke. Fetuses of similar birthweight may vary greatly in their body composition and metabolic capacity, having exhibited different gestational growth trajectories (section 3.2.3).

15. Many determinants of fetal growth are established before conception (section 3.1). A mother's nutritional status at the start of pregnancy influences her ability to meet the demands of her fetus and her baby through dietary intake and nutrient reserves. Ongoing supply is required for a range of nutrients for which there is little reserve in storage.

16. Low maternal status for some micronutrients has some characterised effects on human pregnancy (for example in the case of folate and vitamin D) (section 3.1.4.1.2 and 3.1.4.1.3), but the specific effects of deficiency in many other individual nutrients are currently not well understood.

17   Maternal physiological adaptations normally buffer fetal nutrient supply as maternal nutrient intake fluctuates, but may be insufficient under extreme conditions such as famine. Fetal nutrient supply is then restricted. The stage of gestation at which nutrient supply becomes restricted influences chronic disease risk in a way that can plausibly be related to the sequence of organ and tissue development.

18. After intrauterine growth restriction, the offspring frequently displays an acceleration of early postnatal growth (section 3.4.1). During such "catch-up" (or "compensatory") growth, the relative amounts of tissue deposited may vary from normal. Such disproportionate growth may further alter body composition and metabolic competence, amplifying later disease risk.

19. The type of feeding in infancy also influences the rate of growth and the type of tissue deposited (section 3.5). Infants who are breastfed exhibit a characteristic pattern of growth associated with better health than that observed in infants who are artificially fed. The growth pattern of breastfed infants has therefore been adopted as a "standard" (or desirable) pattern. Early postnatal nutrient exposure can alter hormonal axes and thus has the potential to modify body composition in a way that tracks from fetal life or infancy onwards. These processes may also be influenced by genetic and ethnic variation, although the extent of this is currently not clear.

Observational evidence about the impact of early life nutrition on later chronic disease (Chapter 4)

20.   The largest body of observational evidence considers cardiovascular disease (CVD) outcomes such as coronary heart disease (CHD), and also type 2 diabetes and cancer.

21.   Birthweight is commonly used in observational studies as a proxy for fetal nutritional exposure but it may be influenced by many factors (section 3.2). Birthweight does not sufficiently describe variations in the offspring's body composition or metabolic competencies. Its weakness as an indicator of a newborn's nutritional status at birth deserves wider acknowledgment.

22.   The majority of studies looking at the relationship between birthweight and CHD risk show modest inverse associations: studies of CVD risk factors (blood pressure, serum cholesterol) and birthweight also suggest small inverse associations (section 4.2). Taken together, lower birthweight, lower weight at one year, and increased body mass index (BMI) in childhood are associated with an increased risk of CHD.

23.   Higher birthweight is associated with higher BMI in later life, although there is some doubt about the extent to which this relatively high adult BMI reflects adiposity or muscle mass (section 4.3). The few studies of body composition that have resolved separately the fat and lean mass components suggest that higher birthweight may later be associated with relatively greater lean mass in later life, whereas lower birthweight is associated with relatively greater fat mass. This does not necessarily confirm a direct link between birthweight and central fat distribution.

24.   The evidence suggests that lower birthweight is associated with increased risk of subsequent type 2 diabetes, though there may also be an increased risk at the upper end of the birthweight distribution (section 4.4.1). A rapid increase in adiposity after the age of 2 years is associated with an increased risk of type 2 diabetes in adult life (section 4.4.2).

25.   Greater birthweight is associated with an increased risk of certain cancers in later life, notably breast cancer (particularly in premenopausal women) and child leukaemia (sections 4.5.2.1 and 4.5.1.2). Taller height[i] during childhood and adolescence and more rapid height gain are also associated with an increased risk of premenopausal breast cancer (section 4.5.2.2). Conversely, greater body fatness during childhood and adolescence is associated with a reduced risk of breast cancer (again, particularly premenopausal breast cancer) (section 4.5.2.2).

26.   Overall, the exact relationship between birthweight and later chronic disease risk is complex. The observed relationships vary in strength and consistency; these are not confined to the extremes, and risk tends to be graded across the normal birthweight range. The shape of the association is not clear and does not allow us to define thresholds for healthy birthweight.

---

i   Attained height is often interpreted as a marker for rate of growth.

27. The evidence relating infant feeding practices to subsequent cardiovascular mortality is inconsistent (section 4.2.1.3). However, infants who are not breastfed tend to have slightly higher blood pressure and serum total cholesterol concentrations in adulthood (sections 4.2.2.3 and 4.2.3.2). They may also be at greater risk of type 2 diabetes (section 4.4.3) and are more likely to be obese (i.e. show increased BMI) in later life (section 4.3.3).

28. Higher maternal UVB exposure and circulating 25-hydroxyvitamin D concentrations are associated with greater offspring bone size in later childhood. The relationship with maternal calcium intake or the effects of maternal calcium supplementation are not clear (section 4.6.1). A low rate of childhood growth, particularly in height but also in weight, may also be a risk factor for later hip fracture (section 4.6.3).

29. The review of the epidemiology illustrated how chronic disease outcomes are associated with several indicators of nutritional status in early life. The evidence was reviewed as an illustrative process and predominantly relates to cardiovascular disease, cancer and type 2 diabetes. Consideration of other outcomes would not alter the overall conclusion that variation in nutrient supply during early life is associated with later health outcomes.

30. Although the observational data suggest associations between certain early life exposures and chronic disease outcomes in adulthood, and there is some animal and human evidence to explain underlying mechanisms, it is difficult to detect and quantify meaningful effect sizes for these associations.

Putative mechanisms and their implications (Chapter 5)

31. There is very little human experimental evidence linking long-term outcomes to restriction in the intake of specific nutrients during fetal or early postnatal life. However, observational evidence collected in survivors of famine has shown that the timing of nutrient restriction during gestation, usually severe restriction of both macronutrients and micronutrients, is consistent with the structural and functional effects observed.

32. A few studies have randomly allocated non-breastfed infants to alternative diets. For example, term infants randomly allocated to receive a low sodium diet during the first six months of life showed a lower systolic blood pressure during infancy and adolescence than those receiving a higher sodium diet (section 5.1). Preterm infants randomly allocated to receive donor breastmilk, as opposed to preterm formula, had lower mean and diastolic blood pressure in adolescence. Such studies confirm that early nutrient intake can exert long-term effects on cardiovascular disease risk.

33. In pregnant animal models, limitation of micronutrient or macronutrient intake sufficient to imbalance nutrient supply alters the normal sequence of tissue development (section 5.2). Such modification of phenotype may manifest as change in body weight, size, body composition or function. Each may be altered independently, though there are well-described inter-relationships.

34. Molecular mechanisms can explain how fetal nutrient supply alters phenotype at the cellular and tissue level (section 5.2). For example, animal studies show that imbalanced supply of those nutrients involved in the methylation cycle may induce changes in observable characteristics through epigenetic regulation. The role of epigenetics in human disease is becoming more widely appreciated. Altered · methylation of DNA has been associated with some cancers and atherosclerosis. Epigenetic effects can also account for inter-generational effects observed in animal models.

35. Despite the accumulating animal evidence, no controlled studies in human pregnancy have yet identified maternal dietary interventions that reduce the risk of adult chronic disease in the offspring. Experimental dietary restriction in pregnant animals suggests that the timing, degree and duration of restriction may influence the pattern of fetal development to a greater degree than the choice of nutrient for restriction.

Implications for maternal and child nutrition in the UK (Chapter 6)

36. National studies of diet and nutritional status indicate that excessive consumption of energy from refined carbohydrate and saturated fat, coexists with insufficient intake of vegetables, fruit, and oily fish. In consequence, there is a rising prevalence of obesity, and some evidence of low micronutrient status. These observations raise particular concern about the health of women of reproductive age and young children.

37. Women aged 19-24 years show poor dietary variety and have low intakes of certain micronutrients. Consumption of folic acid supplements remains too low amongst women of childbearing age. There appears to be a lack of awareness of the recommendations to take vitamin D supplements during pregnancy and breastfeeding, and some evidence suggests usage of vitamin D supplements during pregnancy is low, which is of particular concern.

38. There is a lack of national data about the dietary intake and nutritional status of pregnant and breastfeeding women, and of children aged less than 18 months. However, there is some evidence from national surveys that a mother's educational attainment and income predict her dietary choices and infant feeding behaviour.

39. The rising prevalence of obesity in girls and young women represents an important and modifiable risk factor for adverse pregnancy outcome, and for later health outcomes of both the mother and offspring.

Recommendations (Chapter 8)

Public health recommendations

R1 Optimisation of fetal development requires the achievement of adequate nutritional status of the mother prior to conception. Interventions to reduce chronic disease risk in future generations should address dietary and lifestyle change in infancy and adolescence, to ensure adequate nutrition throughout adolescent and reproductive years and in order to improve women's reproductive health.

R2   Efforts to improve diet quality will need to address health inequalities and consider the diet as a whole without neglecting the importance of supplementation with folic acid and vitamin D. Existing advice to increase fruit and vegetable consumption is designed to improve the overall micronutrient status of women along with appropriate folic acid and vitamin D supplementation.

R3   It is particularly important that adolescent and young adult women achieve a body composition and metabolic capacity capable of meeting the stresses of pregnancy as well as their own requirements. This will help to address the health and economic implications of the rising prevalence of maternal obesity for future generations.

R4   There is a need to increase appreciation of the reproductive risks associated with excess maternal body weight and to support women in achieving and maintaining a healthy weight in preparation for pregnancy.

R5   The increased nutritional vulnerability of underweight women needs to be addressed. There is also a need to recognise the increased nutrient demands on adolescent and young women who become pregnant before completing their own growth.

R6   Strategies that promote, protect and support exclusive breastfeeding for around the first six months of an infant's life should be enhanced, and should recognise the benefits for long-term health. The greatest impact is likely to be achieved by intervening in the early postnatal weeks, when the rate of discontinuation is greatest.

Research recommendations

R7   Large, longitudinal cohort studies capable of characterising relationships between early life nutritional exposures and adult chronic disease risk should incorporate measures of pre-conceptional nutritional status, fetal and placental growth, offspring body composition and metabolic competence. Such data will better characterise patterns of pre- and post-natal growth associated with greatest risk of adult chronic disease.

R8   Consideration should be given to building a longitudinal element into national surveys of diet and nutrition in the UK. Repeated measures of body weight and size and dietary intake could be incorporated and linked to health outcome data. The National Diet and Nutrition Survey programme should also consider recruitment of pregnant and breastfeeding women.

R9   Clinical trials investigating changes to the composition of infant formula should incorporate follow-up to capture long-term outcomes.

R10   The causes and consequences of variation in birthweight between ethnic groups need to be better understood, particularly their implications for body composition and metabolic competence. There is an associated need to measure trends in these outcomes as succeeding generations are born in the UK.

R11   Further human research, particularly from intervention studies, is required to understand how maternal body weight and weight gain during pregnancy are related to maternal and offspring health outcome.

R12   Experimental studies in animal models are required to expand understanding of the mechanisms that explain observed associations between nutrition in early life and subsequent chronic disease outcomes. Such studies would help to identify predictive markers of altered function at molecular, cellular, tissue and whole-body level. These phenotypic markers may have application to human studies.

1   Introduction

1. Chronic diseases (such as cardiovascular disease, type 2 diabetes and cancer) are leading causes of death in the UK and thus present a major public health challenge. Many chronic diseases are diet-related. Dietary surveys indicate positive changes in the diet of the UK population but further improvements to the quality and variety of the diet are needed, especially in those groups who are vulnerable, including adolescents and low-income groups. Current nutritional status[ii] has potential implications for the health of future generations [Scientific Advisory Committee on Nutrition, 2008c]. Improving maternal and child nutrition to promote long-term health could also be a driver for future economic growth [World Bank, 2006].

2. Observational studies have reported associations between both over and under nutrition in early life and adult chronic disease. Experimental evidence, principally from animal studies, has offered insight into mechanisms, which may explain and provide plausibility for some of these observations.

3. Support for the concept that maternal, fetal and child nutrition exerts long-term effects and may influence chronic disease risk in adulthood, initially came from ecological studies in Norway where there was considerable variation in cardiovascular mortality rates between different regions. These could not be explained by differences in contemporary living conditions, but were positively associated with earlier infant mortality rates in the same cohorts. Poverty in childhood and adolescence, followed by prosperity, thus appeared to be a risk factor for cardiovascular disease [Forsdahl, 1977; Forsdahl, 1978].

4. Other observations suggest that poverty-related risk factors for chronic disease are modulated through nutrition in fetal life or childhood, and specifically that imbalanced nutrition at a critical stage of development can *programme* the offspring's metabolism in later life [Barker, 1998]. Thus pre- and postnatal factors (including genetic and environmental interactions) could contribute to a phenotype, or phenotypes, that may be more sensitive to lifestyle factors associated with the development of obesity[iii] and chronic disease. This has been labelled the "susceptible phenotype".

5. It is hypothesised that risk of disease in later life increases when there is a difference in relative nutrient supply between the prenatal and postnatal environment. In particular it is argued that risk is increased when the postnatal environment moves

---

ii   The term "nutritional status" is used to describe an individual's position with respect to the maintenance of nutrient homeostasis [Department of Health, 2002]. It is generally assessed by reference to a) energy and nutrient balance, used to estimate the adequacy of dietary supply; b) body size and composition (e.g. body mass index (BMI), waist-hip ratio and more specific estimates of tissue composition and distribution); and c) metabolic and physiological function (e.g. biochemical and dynamic measures of organ and tissue function used to assess the metabolic capacity of an organ or system).

iii In adults, a body mass index (BMI) of >30kg/m². In children, obesity is defined on an age-related basis using a BMI centile that will track to a BMI of 30kg/m² in adulthood. For population monitoring a BMI >95th centile is generally used; for clinical purposes a BMI >98th centile is more commonly cited.

towards high energy intake and low energy expenditure in a population [Hanson & Gluckman, 2005; Gluckman *et al.*, 2010].

6.   Fetal life and early childhood (i.e. up to the age of 5 years) are critical periods for growth and development of an individual, particularly between birth and 2 years of age when nutritional requirements are imposed by rapid growth and development. As children get older, they become less sensitive to external stimuli that may alter their individual phenotype, though adolescence remains important as a time when physical and lifestyle changes affect nutritional needs and eating habits.

7.   Addressing questions about the influence of nutritional exposures at critical time periods, requires an integrated approach that brings together work from both experimental and observational studies (particularly those which examine the relationship of disease risk and birthweight; see section 3.2). This approach, using the totality of the evidence, could shed light on the timing and nature of interventions to improve maternal and child nutrition with long-term benefit.

1.1   Terms of Reference

8.   The Department of Health asked the Scientific Advisory Committee on Nutrition (SACN) to:

• Review the evidence on the influence of maternal, fetal and child nutrition, including growth and development *in utero* and early childhood (i.e. up to the age of 5 years), on the development of chronic disease later in life in the offspring.

• Identify opportunities for nutritional intervention that could influence the risk of chronic disease later in life in the offspring.

9.   The review has been undertaken by SACN's Subgroup on Maternal and Child Nutrition (SMCN). The epidemiological evidence was reviewed in accordance with the principles described in the SACN working document, *A Framework for the Evaluation of Evidence* [Scientific Advisory Committee on Nutrition, 2002].

10.   This report first considers underlying biological concepts related to growth and development of the offspring, particularly the influence of fetal and postnatal nutrient supply (Chapter 3). Epidemiological evidence is then examined and possible confounding factors considered (Chapter 4). Underlying mechanisms are then explored in order to evaluate biological plausibility (Chapter 5). The report finally considers the broader implications of this evidence for maternal and child health, focusing on national surveys of the diet and nutritional status of women and children in the UK (Chapter 6).

11.   SACN originally set out to review chronic disease outcomes, namely cardiovascular disease, diabetes and cancer, where the larger evidence base was at the time. However, SACN recognises that the area of early nutrition and later adult health is a rapidly expanding field. More recently, there has been interest in other areas including allergic diseases, respiratory and dental health, neuro-cognitive function,

mental health behaviour, and muscle strength and function in later life. These may need consideration in the future as the evidence develops.

12.	The Committee has not considered the impact of reproduction on the mother's own later health. Moreover, whilst it recognises that smoking, alcohol and other environmental factors affect development of the offspring, such factors are not considered as primary exposures in this report, only as potential confounders or intermediary factors.

2   Methodological Considerations

13.   SACN initially undertook a systematic review[iv] of the relevant epidemiology published before March 2004. Relevant evidence published since that time has also been considered, until 1st January 2010. The initial systematic review was commissioned to the Division of Community and Health Sciences at St George's, University of London, and helped to stimulate the Committee's discussion. Chapter 4 (*Impact of early nutrition on later chronic disease outcomes: epidemiological studies*) includes the original epidemiological review complemented by further meta-analytical[v] and systematic reviews published since that time (until 1st January 2010).

14.   In the absence of reviews, SACN identified relevant individual retrospective or prospective studies and trials. It then considered experimental studies in humans and animals when exploring mechanistic explanations for the epidemiological observations.

15.   The following section briefly considers methodological issues associated with reviewing the epidemiological evidence, and the strengths and weaknesses of different study designs (see also section 4.1 *Contribution of the epidemiological evidence*).

2.1   Human data

16.   The evidence base in this area is growing, but is largely limited to cohort or cross-sectional studies. Most of the available evidence relates to cardiovascular disease in later life but other outcome measures were considered where sufficient evidence was available. Where systematic reviews or meta-analyses were not available, further literature searches were performed using PubMed, to identify relevant retrospective or prospective studies and trials. SACN did not assess the quality of meta-analyses or systematic reviews and the heterogeneous nature of this evidence obviated the use of standard grading methods (often employed to judge the quality of evidence) applicable to systematic reviews of the human literature.

17.   Experimental studies in humans and animals (see section 2.2 *Reviewing the evidence from animal studies*) were considered when exploring mechanistic explanations for the epidemiological observations.

---

iv   Systematic review – an extensive search for published literature on a specific topic using a defined strategy, with a priori inclusion and exclusion criteria.

v   Meta-analysis – a quantitative pooling of estimates of effect of an exposure on a given outcome, from different studies identified from a systematic review of the literature.

2.1.1   Observational studies

18.   Cohort or cross-sectional observational studies form a major part of the evidence base because the human lifespan imposes long intervals between exposure and outcome. Moreover, the ethical constraints on conducting maternal, fetal and child dietary interventions are considerable. Prospective studies involve follow-up of subjects identified in early life about whom data on a variety of exposures are collected. Because consequences may take years to manifest, such studies often incorporate proxy or intermediate outcome measures that are believed to be indicative of later risk.

19.   Historical (retrospective) cohort studies can yield results more rapidly, and often allow investigation of early life factors and disease end-points (for example, occurrence of, or death from, heart disease). However, the quality of data from pregnancy, infancy and childhood, particularly with nutritional exposures, may be sub-optimal since initial data collection was not intended for this purpose. Additionally these studies often regard size or weight at birth as proxy measures of nutritional exposure during pregnancy and this may not be valid (see section 3.2 *Birthweight*). Finally, the relevance of historical data to contemporary circumstances may also be questioned.

20.   Data collected retrospectively by interview or questionnaire are prone to recall bias. Other exposures during the life course may well confound the relationship between early nutritional influences and later disease outcome; these include social and economic influences, alcohol consumption, smoking uptake, exposure to passive smoking, and physical activity. It is hard to obtain accurate and precise measures for all such confounding factors so that their effects can be accurately quantified or adjusted for in analyses, leading to residual confounding. Factors such as current age, body weight, size, gender and ethnicity can be more readily accounted for in both types of observational studies. Genetic factors could also operate and may predispose both to disease and low birthweight (LBW)[vi].

21.   Historical cohort and prospective cohort data may generate apparent contradictions in the scientific evidence, but this can frequently be attributed to inconsistencies in study design, study population, outcomes and statistical approach. Each design investigates different aspects of the process by which nutritional experience contributes to adult disease risk. This can result in varying emphasis on conclusions reached [Wells, 2009]. Historical cohort studies often demonstrate stronger associations between early life and disease outcomes, whereas modern prospective observational studies have better measures of exposure and confounders. Prospective cohort studies in defined large populations measure them precisely and follow them longitudinally. They are also better able to measure and control or adjust for known confounding factors.

---

vi   Low birthweight (LBW) is defined as a birthweight less than 2.5kg due to being born too early and/or being small for length of gestation (see section 3.2 on *Birthweight*).

22. Meta-analyses and systematic reviews can also be subject to publication bias, which should be considered when identifying and selecting studies for inclusion (see section 4.1.1 *Methodological issues in observational studies*).

2.1.2   Experimental studies

23. Generally, randomised controlled trials (RCTs)[vii] in humans are regarded as methodologically the best approach for studying clinical interventions, but until recently have rarely been applied to investigating the effect of early nutritional exposures on outcomes in later life. The European Union funded Early Nutritional Programming Project (EARNEST) is one collaborative investigation (across 16 countries) into the long-term consequences of early nutrition by metabolic programming. It uses an approach incorporating knowledge from RCTs, epidemiological investigation and animal experimentation (www.metabolic-programming.org).

24. The advantage of RCTs is that known and unknown confounding factors are equally balanced between treatment groups when studies are adequately powered. Hence, the only difference will be in the exposure or treatment of interest, and causation can be directly established. They also allow quantification of the size of effect and help to identify adverse effects, and could inform further benefit analysis. On the other hand; disease outcomes may not become apparent for decades, which necessitates dependence on presumed markers of later disease risk, as are used in prospective cohort studies.

25. RCTs have been conducted in a few specific circumstances in humans, for example following preterm birth [Singhal *et al.*, 2004]. Although the Committee recognise the important biological differences between preterm and term babies, it has considered some data collected from such studies in an attempt to understand some of the causal relationships, which cannot be extracted from epidemiological studies (section 5.1).

26. Follow-up of participants in population-scale, cluster RCTs of early breastfeeding promotion and support, may also provide some evidence of the effects of early feeding on later outcomes [Simell *et al.*, 2000; Kramer *et al.*, 2001]. However, the history of such large-scale interventions is relatively recent.

2.2   Reviewing the evidence from animal studies

27. A great deal of between-study variation exists in some of the human epidemiological literature. Few studies have included direct measures of maternal nutritional status before or during pregnancy on later disease outcomes among offspring. Animal studies allow a greater variety of nutritional interventions than is possible in humans, and enable the controlled investigation of putative mechanisms of nutrition programming. They also allow identification of the precise developmental windows in which early nutritional imbalances can contribute to later disease. Thus,

---

vii Randomised controlled trial (RCT) – a study in which eligible participants are assigned to two or more treatment groups on a random allocation basis. Randomisation assures the play of chance so that all sources of bias, known and unknown, are equally balanced between treatment groups.

the contributions of human and animal research can be complementary, despite the problems of inter-species extrapolation, which are particularly relevant to the reproductive period [Symonds, 2007].

28.　　Animal studies provide a body of evidence to support the hypothesis that prenatal nutrient supply, encountered within the physiological range of variation, programmes disease risk in later life. Studies in animals looking at possible molecular and cellular mechanisms that lead to changes in physiology are considered later in Chapter 5. Exposing the developing rat or sheep fetus to only moderate maternal food restriction, or restricting the supply of specific nutrients, results in altered physiology and the initiation of disease processes [Bertram & Hanson, 2001; Langley-Evans, 2001]. Dietary manipulations in animal models are, however, sometimes extreme, and extrapolating to consequences for humans is not always easy or appropriate.

3   Background

29.   Growth and development involve a series of changes by which the fetus becomes a mature organism. This amounts to much more than simply the addition of cells and tissues to achieve an increase in body mass. Changes include a specialisation of various parts of the body to perform different functions, and alterations in the form of the body as a whole, as well as in the form of individual organs and systems [Sinclair, 1989].

30.   Normal growth and development is therefore characterised by a regulated increase in the size, mass *and* complexity of function of tissues and organs. Thus, differential growth and development during fetal life and early childhood could lead to differences in body composition and metabolic and physiological function, and influence chronic disease risk in adulthood.

31.   A distinction has been made in this report between the terms "size" and "weight". "Size" denotes linear dimensions (such as length, height and head circumference) whereas "weight" is used to describe body mass. Explicit reference has been made to measures such as body mass index (BMI) or ponderal index[viii] (measures of body weight which adjust for height) where relevant.

32.   Growth and development is absolutely dependant on a supply of energy and nutrients sufficient to match the variable need as growth progresses [Jackson, 1996]. Any limitation of supply is likely to constrain the pace and pattern of development [Wootton & Jackson, 1995]. The pattern of growth has a characteristic tempo, which can be disturbed if nutrient intake is inadequate or excessive, or if disease impairs nutrient uptake and utilisation. The measurement of growth, therefore, is a key tool for monitoring fetal, infant and child health (see section 3.5 *Influences on growth*).

33.   In functional terms, growth represents a progressive increase in metabolic capacity, and maturity marks the acquisition of the full adult capacity [Jackson, 1996]. The ability of individuals to adapt and cope with a wide range of environments and stressors, reflects a reserve capacity. A constraint on growth and development, imposed by nutritional limitation at a critical stage of development, can have a substantial effect on the acquisition of capacity [Langley-Evans, 2004].

34.   Some basic underlying concepts relating to pre and postnatal growth and development are outlined in the following sections, and the role nutrition plays during these processes is described. The chapter also describes how early life experiences can determine causes and timing of mortality.

---

viii   Ponderal Index (PI) is an index of fatness, often used as a measure of obesity – the body weight in kilograms divided by the length in meters cubed (kg/m³).

3.1 Fetal growth

35. Fetal growth and development is a highly organised process in which complex changes are coordinated sequentially in time, and changes at the molecular and cellular level are integrated to enable development of the whole organism [World Health Organization, 2006]. Immediately after fertilisation takes place, cell division begins and progresses at a rapid rate.

36. Embryogenesis is the process confined to the first trimester by which the embryo is formed and develops. It starts with the fertilisation of the ovum (egg); rapid mitotic divisions and cellular differentiation then lead to development of an embryo. During this time, the developing embryo is sensitive to environmental factors. As the fertilized egg begins to divide, organ structure and function begin to develop. The fetal period begins 10 weeks after the first day of the last menstrual period (8 weeks after fertilisation), and by this time the precursors of all the major organs of the body have been created.

37. Once the placenta is fully established, fetal development is dependent on the integrity of the maternal-placental unit. Severely disrupted placental function can impair the delivery of nutrients and oxygen to the fetus and constrain fetal growth. Fetal growth is also heavily influenced by maternal stress and workload, the mother's metabolic capacity, and her general health [World Health Organization, 2006].

3.1.1 Determinants of fetal growth

38. Genetic, epigenetic and environmental factors influence fetal (and postnatal) growth, and the progress of any infant's development is the result of a complex interaction of many factors. Maternal weight at first antenatal-clinic visit, maternal height, length of gestation, sex, parity and ethnicity are all determinants of birthweight [Gardosi et al., 1992] (see section 3.2 Birthweight); as are pathological factors such as smoking [Lumley et al., 2000], alcohol abuse [Little & Wendt, 1991] and pregestational or gestational diabetes [Weintrob et al., 1996]. Paternal height has also been shown to be positively associated with offspring size at birth [Morrison et al., 1991; Wilcox et al., 1995; Godfrey et al., 1997; Veena et al., 2004 Harvey et al., 2008], suggesting potential genetic influences on skeletal growth.

39. Maternal constraint, by which maternal and uteroplacental factors act to limit the growth of the fetus, is an important physiological cause of the variation in birth size [Gluckman & Hanson, 2004]. Maternal constraint acts in all pregnancies, but the influence is greater in some situations, for example with small maternal size as classically shown by crossing reciprocally a large Shire horse and a small Shetland pony. The pair in which the mother was the Shire had a large newborn foal, and the pair in which the mother was Shetland had a small foal. After a few months, both foals were the same size (see section 3.4.1 Canalisation, catch-up and catch down growth), and attained an adult size half-way between their parents [Walton & Hammond, 1938].

40. Similarly in human pregnancies, after ovum donation, small women tend to have babies with lower birthweight, even when the woman donating the egg is large [Brooks *et al.*, 1995]. The growth of the fetus is thought to be constrained towards the end of pregnancy in order that the mother can achieve successful delivery; twins slow down earlier when their combined weight is approximately the weight of a 36 week singleton fetus [Tanner, 1990].

41. Infant birthweight is also correlated with the mother's own birthweight and with that of other female relatives [Shah & Shah, 2009]. Women who were born of low birthweight were more likely than their non-LBW counterparts to deliver offspring with LBW [Coutinho *et al.*, 1997; Shah & Shah, 2009]. It is unclear whether this constraining mechanism is related to maternal diet.

42. Maternal supply of nutrients needs to accord with fetal demand in order to achieve healthy growth and development of the fetus, thus avoiding potential consequences for long-term health [Constancia *et al.*, 2005]. Although the mother has some ability to adapt to ensure a supply of nutrients to the fetus, her dietary supply remains important. Interdependency between nutrients emphasises the importance of dietary balance: for example, supply of micronutrients may alter the way in which macronutrients are utilised for energy [Herrera, 2000].

3.1.2 Metabolic anticipation in pregnancy

43. Pregnancy involves major anatomical, physiological, and metabolic changes in the mother to support and provide for the needs of both the growing fetus and herself [Catalano *et al.*, 1998; Jackson, 2000; Duggleby & Jackson, 2002a; von Versen Hoeynck & Powers, 2007].

44. Successful pregnancy requires the net deposition of tissue within the mother, the placenta and the fetus, and complex metabolic changes take place at different times during pregnancy to support the changing needs of the developing fetus. Metabolic anticipation occurs, where these changes occur in advance of fetal demand. Thus changes in maternal nitrogen metabolism anticipate the later needs of the fetus [Duggleby & Jackson, 2002a]. In addition, maternal fat deposition during pregnancy anticipates the requirements for fetal growth in the last quarter of gestation [Sohlstrom & Forsum, 1995]. Pregnancy liberates nutrients from body stores as the blood supply to the fetoplacental unit increases; these changes begin to occur at the earliest stages of the pregnancy, well before fetal demands can form a significant proportion of the mother's nutritional balance. However, an ongoing supply of nutrients to the mother is required, particularly for some nutrients for which there is little reserve in storage.

45. In some circumstances, maternal dietary supply may not meet fetal demand. For example, the dietary supply of docosohexaenoic acid (22:6 *n-3*; DHA) may not balance the high rate of utilisation associated with growth of the fetal brain in late pregnancy. In these circumstances, the placenta plays an important role in mobilising fatty acids from maternal adipose tissue stores deposited earlier and actively selecting the *n-3* and *n-6* fatty acids for uptake and retention [Haggarty, 2004].

46. Adaptive processes thus operate to maintain a degree of constancy in fetal nutrient supply, buffering the fetal cellular microenvironment from the usual unevenness of dietary intake. This capability could itself be in part a programmed metabolic capability, with the specific maternal phenotype determined by the mother's nutritional environment in her own fetal and early postnatal life, when the opportunity for moulding metabolic plasticity still exists [Jackson, 2005].

3.1.3   Fetal nutrient supply

47. Adequate nutrient supply to the fetus is crucial to the attainment of normal growth, maturation and bone mineral accretion. Increased maternal food consumption, elevated gastrointestinal absorption, decreased or increased mineral excretion and mobilisation of tissue stores are complementary strategies that can contribute to meet increased requirements, particularly with respect to bone-forming minerals. Pregnancy is associated with physiological changes in mineral metabolism that are independent of maternal mineral supply within the range of normal dietary intakes. In a well-nourished woman, these processes, amongst others, can provide the bone-forming minerals necessary for fetal growth without requiring an increase in dietary intake [Prentice, 2003].

48. Both the fetus and the exclusively breastfed infant are totally dependent on the mother's ability to transfer nutrients at the appropriate time. The mother's ability to achieve effective and timely transfer is constrained by factors other than her immediate dietary intake or overall nutritional status.

49. The fetal nutrient 'supply line' [Harding, 2001] incorporates several interconnected and coordinated steps (see Figure 1), which collectively satisfy fetal demands regardless of the current dietary intake of the mother. The mother has the ability to draw on her nutrient reserves as and when necessary to satisfy this changing pattern of demands. The female offspring's own subsequent development towards achievement of metabolic capacity, will in turn determine her own capability for successful pregnancy, and may thus have intergenerational consequences.

Figure 1 – Intergenerational aspects of maternal, fetal and infant nutrition on development and predisposition to disease risk. The diagram illustrates how environmental factors and diet (purple boxes) modify nutritional status throughout the reproductive cycle. Maternal considerations are shown in yellow; placental considerations in green; fetal in blue and offspring in orange.

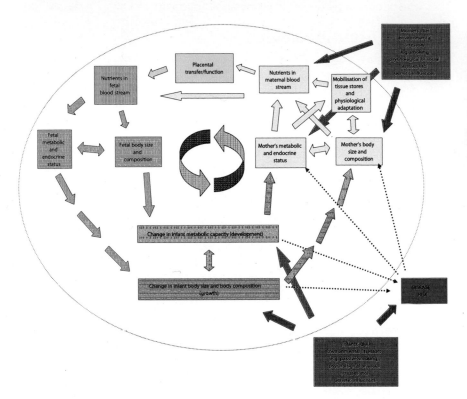

50. Endocrine signals are received and transmitted between the mother and fetus through the placenta, and this is the site of nutrient exchange. The placenta influences substrate flow and has an important role in regulating fetal growth and development by modulating the fetal endocrine milieu, e.g. insulin-like growth factor (IGF) axes of the fetus, placenta and mother. Umbilical blood flow and fetal endocrine status then regulate the uptake of nutrients by the fetus. Adequate placental function is a prerequisite for fetal growth which can be impaired if perfusion of the placental bed is reduced, for example by maternal pre-eclampsia, in spite of adequate maternal nutrient supply [Murphy *et al.*, 2006].

51. Various aspects of disrupted placental function, including altered morphology, blood flow and fetal oxygen supply, can alter the capacity for exchange of nutrients between the mother and the fetus, thereby being a major cause of fetal growth abnormalities [Sibley *et al.*, 2005; Sibley, 2009].

52. Placental failure has been implicated as a cause of poor fetal nutrition [Garnica & Chan, 1996], leading to changes in body weight, size and composition at birth. Studies of fetal nutrient supply, employing techniques such as cordocentesis (umbilical blood sampling *in utero*), have emphasised the importance of placental function as a determinant of fetal growth restriction [Pardi & Cetin, 2006].

53.	Changes may be more subtle than reduction in birthweight. For example, the ratio of placental weight to fetal weight has been related to the rate of postnatal growth. Babies born small but with a relatively large placenta, are less likely to show catch-up growth[ix] (see section 3.4.1) in the 18 months after birth [Harding & McCowan, 2003]. The authors' interpretation of this was that failure to show catch-up growth after birth, suggests that such babies are affected by an intrinsic growth defect rather than an extrinsic limitation by the intrauterine environment.

54.	For a well-nourished population of women, the pattern of food intake may relate less well to birth outcomes than the nutritional status of the mother at conception and her capacity to achieve extensive metabolic interchange [Duggleby & Jackson, 2002b; Jackson et al., 2003]. The imposition of any stress is likely to alter nutritional state, either by changing appetite, changing the partitioning of nutrients between tissues, increasing nutrient losses, or altering the pattern of demand for nutrients [Jackson et al., 2003].

55.	These factors include the broader stresses imposed by society, and the life choices that are available to the mother. Stresses such as infection or inflammatory challenges, high workload, psychological or social stresses, and cigarette smoking, can impose further nutritional demands that alter the handling of nutrients within the body and their availability to the tissues [Jackson et al., 2003]. Deprivation in pregnancy, defined by factors such as income, employment, housing, education and skills, is also shown to increase the risk of preterm birth and is associated with diets low in protein, fibre, minerals and vitamins [Haggarty et al, 2009].

56	Glucose is the principal fetal fuel. In the presence of maternal euglycaemia (normal blood glucose concentration) and normal placental function the transplacental supply meets fetal glucose requirements. Glucose is transported across the placenta in proportion to its concentration in the maternal circulation and according to the rate of placental blood flow. Placental and fetal gluconeogenesis, especially from amino acids, occurs in the ovine and human and may be particularly important during fetal hypoglycaemia.

57.	Maternal plasma glucose originates from both dietary and endogenous sources, principally the liver. Dietary energy is stored by the mother as fat in the first half of pregnancy; greater insulin sensitivity is thought to be the stimulus [Boden, 1996; Knopp, 1997; Herrera, 2000]. By the third trimester, increasing insulin resistance triggers the lipolysis of stored fat, and the release of free fatty acids from those stores. Free fatty acids are an alternative metabolic fuel for the mother and help to conserve glucose supply to the fetus [Scholl et al., 2001]. Glucose uptake in maternal liver and muscle are reduced and hepatic glucose production increased [Homko et al., 1999]. After 30 weeks gestation, a modest net loss of maternal body fat occurs [Hytten, 1974] and this net mobilisation corresponds with an exponential increase in fetal fat during which 94% of all fat deposition in the fetus occurs [Widdowson, 1968].

---

ix	Catch-up growth is rapid growth following a period of restriction. Ultimately, it may redress wholly or partly the accrued deficit in weight or size though there may be consequences for body composition and metabolic capacity.

58. Several studies have found that women following diets composed of low glycaemic index (GI) foods were more likely to have infants who were small for gestational age (SGA)[x] and of lower birthweight [Clapp, III, 2002; Scholl et al., 2004]. This may reflect the energy density of different GI diets and thus total energy intake, and subsequent effects on maternal weight gain and infant birthweight. A dietary intervention study found that infants of women assigned to foods of moderate to high GI were heavier than those eating foods of low GI [Moses et al., 2006]. Infants in the former group had a higher ponderal index (PI) too. Other studies have reported inverse associations between carbohydrate intake and birthweight [Godfrey et al., 1996] and 'total sugar' intake[xi] and birthweight [Lenders et al., 1994].

59. The placenta plays multiple roles in ensuring the balance of nutrient delivery from mother to fetus. This is critical for the delivery of amino acids to the fetus and in the removal of the end products of fetal metabolism, such as urea. The pattern of amino acids required by the fetus for net tissue deposition, gluconeogensis and regulatory metabolic function, requires significant modulation of that present in blood. This appears to be particularly important for the delivery to the fetus of conditionally essential amino acids such as serine/glycine and glutamine/arginine, which are thought to be critically limiting for normal pregnancy, as sufficient supply through endogenous pathways appears marginal for the demands.

3.1.4 Effect of variation in maternal nutritional status on birthweight and size

60. There is a complex metabolic interplay between the competing needs of the fetus and those of the mother. The mother may have her own demands for nutrients that compete with the needs of the fetus, especially in the case of the teenage mother still completing her own growth [Scholl et al., 1994]. It is important to acknowledge the role of nutrient supply from conception, which in turn requires that the nutritional status of the mother is capable of fuelling a fetus throughout her reproductive years [Ozanne & Hales, 2004; World Health Organization, 2005].

3.1.4.1 Maternal diet

61. Physiological mechanisms in the mother buffer fetal nutrient supply when there is restriction in maternal diet. The success of these mechanisms determines the effect of nutrient and energy restriction on fetal outcome. Where there is chronic maternal energy or nutrient deficiency, these mechanisms may not be robust and the fetal substrate supply may become insufficient, slowing fetal growth. This was observed in an intervention study performed in The Gambia [Ceesay et al., 1997].

---

x   Small-for-gestational-age (SGA) is defined as a newborn whose weight falls below a given threshold (most commonly <10th percentile) on a specified birthweight reference.

xi The term "total sugar", as defined by the author, refers to the sum of simple carbohydrates, including monosaccharides (i.e. galactose, glucose, mannose, fructose), disaccharides (i.e. lactose, sucrose, maltose), and oligosaccharides (i.e. ribose, xylose) which are naturally occurring in foods or are added to manufactured foods. It does not include any complex carbohydrate such as starch or fibre.

3.1.4.1.1   Macronutrients

62.   Studies of pregnancies occurring during the Dutch famine of 1944-1945 found that mothers with severely restricted energy and nutrient intakes during late gestation tended to bear smaller offspring [Stein *et al.*, 2004]. Measures of birthweight, crown-to-heel length and head circumference, all declined with famine exposure late in pregnancy (see later section 3.4.2 *Critical periods and programming in humans*).

63.   A Cochrane review of trials on the impact of increased maternal energy and protein intake during pregnancy, in mainly undernourished populations, showed that balanced energy/protein supplementation was associated with modest increases in maternal weight gain and in mean birthweight, and a substantial reduction in risk of small for gestational age birth [Kramer & Kakuma, 2003]. In contrast, protein supplementation during pregnancy was associated with an increased risk of small for gestational age birth. The UK trials included in the review that showed a small effect were conducted among nutritionally "at risk" mothers [Elwood *et al.*, 1981; Viegas *et al.*, 1982]. Overall, the review reported a mean increase in birthweight of only 37 g at term. One explanation may be that women who were entered into the trials because of concern about longstanding nutritional status, received the intervention too late, with the fetal growth trajectory having been set much earlier in gestation [Bloomfield *et al.*, 2006].

3.1.4.1.2   Folate

64.   It is well recognised that low folate status is associated with an increased risk of neural tube defects (NTD) which can be reduced by increasing the periconceptional intake of folic acid [Department of Health, 2000; Scientific Advisory Committee on Nutrition, 2006].

65.   The results obtained in many, but not all [de Weerd *et al.*, 2003], observational studies have suggested that low folate intake or low circulating folate concentration in pregnancy is associated with increased risk of preterm delivery and low birthweight [Scholl & Johnson, 2000; Relton *et al.*, 2005; Tamura & Picciano, 2006; Torrens *et al.*, 2006].

66.   Rao *et al.*, (2001) observed a positive association between birthweight and dietary intake of folate-rich foods in rural Indian women. Furthermore, birthweight and maternal red blood cell folate status were positively correlated at 28 weeks gestation [Rao *et al.*, 2001]. A prospective cohort study observed that pregnant adolescents with low folate intake, as well as those with low red cell and serum folate, were significantly more likely to deliver a small for gestational age baby [Baker *et al.*, 2009].

67.   A prospective cohort of pregnant women from the Amsterdam Born Children and their Development study (ABCD) suggested that folate status may be relevant only when the folate status of the mother at conception is low. At short interpregnancy intervals (i.e. <6 months), women who did not take folic acid supplements were found to be at greater risk of fetal growth restriction (as reflected by lower mean birthweight and higher SGA risk) [van Eijsden *et al.*, 2008b].

68. However, a prospective cohort study, in a different population, examining the links between deprivation and diet in pregnancy found no link between folate status and birth outcome [Haggarty et al., 2009]. Results from randomised controlled trials with folic acid have also not supported an effect [Scholl & Johnson, 2000; Charles et al., 2005]. It has also been argued that any connection between low folate status and birth outcome, may in fact be attributable to maternal obesity, which is associated with poorer folate status [Prentice & Goldberg, 1996; Rasmussen et al., 2008].

69. The link between maternal folate status and offspring birthweight is, therefore, unclear, especially in the context of a relatively well-nourished population. There is no information from human studies about the effect of the mother's folate intake on body composition or metabolic competence of the offspring.

3.1.4.1.3 Vitamin D

70. Vitamin-D deficiency rickets[xii], a disorder that becomes apparent during infancy or childhood, is the result of insufficient amounts of vitamin D in the body. This impairs the absorption of dietary calcium and phosphorus resulting in poor mineralisation of the skeleton [Holick, 2006]. Observational studies provide evidence for a role of vitamin D in prenatal bone development (see section 4.6 *Bone mineral density and bone mass*).

71. Adequate circulating concentrations of 25-hydroxyvitamin D (the main circulating vitamin D metabolite) during pregnancy are necessary to ensure appropriate maternal responses to the calcium demands of the fetus and neonatal handling of calcium [Specker, 2004]. It is essential that women entering pregnancy achieve an adequate vitamin D status to ensure supply to the fetus and thus the infant during the early months of life [Scientific Advisory Committee on Nutrition, 2007b].

72. Seasonal variation in birthweight has been observed, with babies born in October being slightly heavier than those born in May. It has been speculated that this reflects variation in vitamin D status attributable to differences in sunlight exposure [McGrath et al., 2005], though other seasonal influences such as weight gain in winter, and fruit and vegetable intake in summer, may be operative. A study in The Gambia, where there is tropical UVB sunlight exposure all year round, observed no significant relationships between maternal vitamin D status and birthweight [Prentice et al., 2009].

73. A Canadian prospective study of pregnant women who were low milk consumers, observed a positive association between birthweight and milk consumption [Mannion et al., 2006]. This was attributed to greater vitamin D intake (cow's milk is fortified with vitamin D in Canada) but differences in the intake of other milk constituents, such as protein, might equally be responsible.

74. Several studies in developed countries where cow's milk is not fortified with vitamin D have investigated the relationship between maternal consumption of cow's milk during pregnancy and birthweight. The results have been equivocal

---

xii Rickets – malformation of the skeleton in growing children due to osteomalacia (softening of the bones).

[Elwood *et al.*, 1981; Godfrey *et al.*, 1996; Ludvigsson & Ludvigsson, 2004; Mitchell *et al.*, 2004; Moore *et al.*, 2004], but a large prospective study in Denmark (n=50,117 mother-infant pairs) observed that maternal milk consumption in mid-pregnancy was inversely associated with the risk of small-for gestational age at birth, and positively associated with both large-for gestational age at birth and mean birthweight (P_{trend}=0.001) [Olsen *et al.*, 2007]. It was suggested that the protein intake from cow's milk was related to birthweight, but the role of dietary calcium was not evaluated due to high collinearity of milk and total dietary calcium intakes.

3.1.4.1.4 Long chain polyunsaturated fatty acids (PUFA) – n-3 fatty acids

75. SACN previously reviewed trials in Europe and the US investigating maternal dietary supplementation with long chain *n-3* polyunsaturated fatty acids (LC *n-3* PUFA) [Scientific Advisory Committee on Nutrition, 2004]. It was noted that trials showing effects on increased gestation length [Olsen *et al.*, 1992; Smuts *et al.*, 2003], and reduced preterm delivery [Olsen *et al.*, 2000], tended to be in 'at risk' populations or those with lower mean birthweight. In trials showing no effect of maternal LC *n-3* PUFA supplementation on infant birthweight or gestation, the mean birthweight of the control group exceeded 3600g [Helland *et al.*, 2001; Malcolm *et al.*, 2003]. The effect of *n-3* fatty acid supplementation may also be affected by the pattern of fish consumption before and during pregnancy which potentially alters the balance of long chain PUFA released from maternal stores during pregnancy [Scientific Advisory Committee on Nutrition, 2004].

76. A meta-analysis of RCTs of women with "low-risk" pregnancies concluded that LC *n-3* PUFA supplementation during pregnancy may enhance pregnancy duration and infant head circumference, but the mean effect size was small [Szajewska *et al.*, 2006]. A systematic review of RCTs of women with "high-risk" pregnancies observed that LC *n-3* PUFA supplementation during pregnancy was associated with reduced risk of delivery before 34 weeks of gestation (relative risk (RR) 0.39, 95% confidence interval (CI) 0.18, 0.84). However, there was no effect on mean birthweight, gestation, risk of delivery before 37 weeks or incidence of low birthweight [Horvath *et al.*, 2007].

77. The ABCD cohort study found that birthweight was positively associated with plasma *n-3* fatty acid concentrations. In addition, a positive association was observed with the *n-6* fatty acid, dihomo-γ-linolenic acid (DGLA; 20:3 *n-6*), the precursor of arachidonic acid. Negative associations were observed with all other *n-6* fatty acids. These associations were confined to the extremes of exposure, but suggest that a maternal plasma fatty acid profile characterised by low *n-3* and high *n-6* fatty acid concentrations in early pregnancy is associated with reduced fetal growth [van Eijsden *et al.*, 2008a].

3.1.4.1.5 Nutrient interactions

78. The Pune Maternal Nutrition Study (in India) investigated possible associations between maternal nutrition and the offspring's risk of diabetes and heart disease in

later life. This study, conducted in a population with low vitamin B_{12} status, found no association between maternal serum vitamin B_{12} concentration and birthweight or length though fat mass was greatest in the offspring of mothers with highest red blood cell folate concentrations [Yajnik et al., 2008]. High folate status in mothers with the lowest vitamin B_{12} concentrations was particularly associated with insulin resistance in the offspring at 6 years of age. It was suggested that an intrauterine imbalance between these two micronutrients, which are both implicated in methyl group provision might be responsible. A further report suggested that low maternal methylmalonic acid concentrations at 28 weeks predicted low birthweight [Yajnik et al., 2005].

3.1.4.2   Maternal body composition and metabolism

79.   Maternal height, weight and body composition may relate to the metabolic capacity of the mother and thus her ability to deliver nutrients to the fetus.

80.   Maternal obesity has been defined as having a BMI over 30 at first booking [Heslehurst et al., 2007]. Maternal obesity and gestational diabetes are independently associated with increased birthweight and adolescent risk of obesity in the offspring [Langer et al., 2005]. Maternal diabetes (type 1 and 2) and gestational diabetes have also been associated with an increased risk of obesity in offspring both in childhood and adulthood [Wells et al., 2007a].

81.   Maternal pre-pregnancy weight and the weight gained during pregnancy have been associated with the offspring's birthweight [Abrams & Laros, 1986; Kramer, 1987; Scholl et al., 1991; Thame et al., 1997; Abrams et al., 2000]. A retrospective analysis in the UK of 287,213 completed singleton pregnancies, observed that maternal obesity results in offspring who are more likely to have birthweights above the 90th percentile, as well as other complications [Sebire et al., 2001]; this has also been observed elsewhere [Catalano & Ehrenberg, 2006].

82.   Obese women are at significantly increased risk of gestational hypertension, pre-eclampsia and gestational diabetes [Weiss et al., 2004]. Gestational diabetes can develop in the second half of pregnancy and if not controlled leads to excessive transfer of glucose from mother to fetus, inducing fetal hyperglycaemia. This alters fetal pancreatic structure and function leading to increased fetal insulin secretion and macrosomia (the Pedersen hypothesis; Pedersen, 1954; Pedersen, 1977). Women who are obese [Ray et al., 2005] or have pre-gestational diabetes [Correa et al., 2008] are also more likely to have babies with congenital malformations including neural tube defects (NTD).

83.   Maternal obesity is associated with a greater plasma volume and increased placental transfer. It is also associated with a relative increase in maternal insulin resistance, making more glucose available to the fetus [Goldenberg & Tamura, 1996]. During a 3-hour glucose tolerance test in pregnant women, the area under the curve following administration of 50g glucose was significantly correlated with BMI [Green et al., 1990]. Non-fasting maternal glucose concentration also shows a positive association with pre-pregnancy BMI and the summed maternal triceps and subscapular skinfold thickness [Scholl et al., 2001].

84.   In maternal diabetes, these changes are amplified and higher concentrations of maternal glucose and other metabolic fuels (triglycerides, amino acids, free fatty acids, ketones) are transported to the fetus [Boden, 1996; Knopp, 1997; Herrera, 2000]. Third trimester blood glucose levels in diabetic mothers predicted infant birthweight, even after adjustment for smoking and body mass index [Jovanovic-Peterson et al., 1991].

85.   A positive association between third-trimester non-fasting maternal glucose and infant birthweight was observed in non-diabetic women [Scholl et al., 2001]. In addition, high glucose concentrations were associated with a two-fold or more increase in complications such as caesarean section and chorioamnionitis with preterm delivery. These findings were replicated in another American cohort of diabetes-free pregnant women from varied ethnic backgrounds [Scholl et al., 2002].

86.   Newborn infants of women with gestational diabetes show significantly increased fat mass and percent body fat compared to those born to women with normal glucose tolerance; follow-up studies also suggest an increased risk of childhood obesity [Catalano & Ehrenberg, 2006; Wells, 2007]. Another study observed a positive association between childhood obesity (as defined by BMI) at 5-7 years and the mother's plasma glucose levels during pregnancy [Hillier et al., 2007].

87.   Maternal adiposity, as reflected by BMI, is influenced by parity. Greater increases with age are seen among nulliparous or multiparous women than those who have only one or two pregnancies [Brown et al., 1992]. Increasing maternal parity in the Pune Maternal Nutrition Study was associated with greater birthweight, skinfold thickness, and abdominal circumference in the offspring. This relationship was independent of other maternal characteristics [Joshi et al., 2005].

88.   A prospective study conducted in Jamaica found a significant increase in weight and lean body mass gained in pregnancy among adolescent girls compared to mature women [Thame et al., 2007]. This and other studies [Steven-Simons et al., 1993; Jones et al., 2009] suggest that the weight of lean mass gained by an adolescent mother during pregnancy is a strong determinant of infant birthweight. Generally adolescent girls tend to have smaller babies, as observed in a retrospective study of pregnant women in Jamaica [Thame et al., 1999].

3.2   Birthweight

89.   Birthweight is an important indicator of neonatal and perinatal risk. It has been commonly adduced as a summary index of fetal nutritional exposure in epidemiological studies. However, it is now widely recognised that birthweight is neither a sensitive or specific measure of fetal nutrient supply, nor the only measure indicative of fetal nutritional exposure.

90.   *Low birthweight* (LBW) is defined internationally as a birthweight less than 2.5kg. This may be attributable to being born too early, being born small for length of gestation, or both. A *small-for-gestational age* (SGA) baby is one whose birthweight

is below the 10th (or sometimes 3rd) centile weight for estimated gestation. *"Large-for-gestational age"* refers to babies whose birthweight exceeds the 90th centile.

3.2.1 Birthweight distribution

91. The frequency distribution of birthweights has two components, being composed of a predominant bell-shaped curve with an extended lower tail. An example of this is given in Figure 2, which shows the birthweight distribution of a population similar to that of the UK. The 'predominant' distribution, defined by its mean and standard deviation (SD), covers the majority of births and corresponds closely with the birthweight distribution of term babies. The lower tail of the curve, the 'residual' distribution, comprises all births that fall outside the predominant distribution and typically amounts to 2-5% of all births. Not all preterm births fall within this residual distribution; it is only the smallest births, which happen to also be those at highest perinatal risk. Populations with a larger proportion in the lower tail end would therefore be expected to have a greater number of small preterm births, and in turn, a higher infant mortality rate. A small excess of large births in the upper tail of the distribution includes babies of diabetic and prediabetic mothers whose increased growth rate is also associated with higher than average morbidity and mortality [Wilcox, 2001].

Figure 2 – Distribution of birthweights for 405,676 live and still births, Norway, 1992–1998 [Wilcox, 2001]

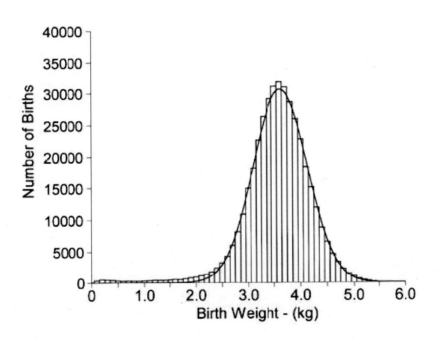

Reproduced from: Wilcox AJ, On the importance – and the unimportance – of birth weight. Int J Epidemiol 2001, vol 30, pages 1233-1241, with permission from Oxford University Press.

92.	The average birthweight varies in different populations, as does the optimal birthweight (the weight associated with the lowest perinatal mortality) [Wilcox & Russell, 1986; Graafmans *et al.*, 2002]. A study analysing data from the nationally representative UK Millenium Cohort Study (n=16,157) reported mean birthweight in the white infants to be 3.42 kg (95% CI 3.40, 3.43 kg) (unadjusted) [Kelly *et al.*, 2008].

### 3.2.2	Secular trends in birthweight

93.	In most industrialised countries over the last twenty years, there has been a secular trend of increasing birthweight [Cole, 2000]. The pace of the trend might be attributable more to rising maternal weight than height [Cole, 2003].

94.	In contrast, since the 1970s there has been an increase in the proportion of low birthweight babies reported in Japan. This has been associated with decreasing maternal BMI, reflecting the cosmetic concerns of younger women, and the increasing prevalence of smoking [Ohmi *et al.*, 2001].

95.	In the UK, average birthweight and the risk of low birthweight differs substantially between ethnic groups [Harding *et al.*, 2004; Tate *et al.*, 2006; Kelly *et al.*, 2008] (see Chapter 6).

96.	Maternal birthweight and adult height are likely to be influenced by the health and social and economic change across generations [Haggarty *et al*, 2009]. Intergenerational effects on birthweight have been observed (see earlier section *3.1.1 Determinants of fetal growth*); a mother who was herself of low birthweight is twice as likely to have LBW offspring [Shah & Shah, 2009] (see section 3.4.2 *Critical periods and programming in humans*).

### 3.2.3	Limitations of birthweight as an indicator of phenotype

97.	Although birthweight provides some information about the end point of fetal growth, it neither describes the fetal growth trajectory nor reflects body composition. The pattern of fetal growth may affect the development of organs and physiologic systems in ways that are not predicted by birthweight and body proportions [Prentice & Goldberg, 2000]. Birthweight alone is therefore a relatively insensitive measure of fetal nutritional status and may be best regarded as an "outcome of convenience" for perinatal health policy [Wilcox, 2001] rather than a complete descriptor of nutritional phenotype.

98.	Birthweight is also subject to other influences, including environmental contaminants and, importantly, the mother's physique and parity. For example, smoking during pregnancy increases the risk of low birthweight and preterm delivery [Lumley *et al.*, 1998].

99.	Babies are frequently categorised as "small" or "large" for gestational age on the basis of their birthweight but this approach is problematic. Firstly, epidemiological data indicate a gradation of metabolic risk across the birthweight range. Secondly, adjustment of birthweight for maternal characteristics leads to reclassification of substantial numbers of babies as "small" or "large" [Gardosi *et al.*, 1992].

Thirdly, birthweight and other body proportions are normally distributed within populations [Kramer *et al.*, 1989].

100. Measures of size and body composition at birth are recorded much less frequently and often less precisely than birthweight which is routinely captured in clinical records. Hence, associations with parameters other than weight have been less systematically examined in historic cohort studies.

3.3 Postnatal growth

101. The average length of human pregnancy is 280 days, or 40 weeks, from the first day of the mother's last menstrual period, but there is considerable variation in length across the range of 37 to 42 completed weeks of gestation. Babies born within these limits are 'term' babies; whereas, those born before are 'preterm' and those born after 'post-term'. Some of the variation in the timing of birth relates to differences in the period between last menstrual period and subsequent ovulation/conception.

102. During pre- and postnatal growth, energy is required for the synthesis of growing tissues. The proportion of energy intake utilised for growth is highest in the first 3 months after birth when it accounts for about 35% of the total energy requirement for the average term infant (and this is higher for infants born preterm). This proportion is halved in the next three months (i.e. to approximately 17.5%), and further reduced to only 3% at 12 months (Figure 3) [Wells & Davies 1998]. Energy needs for growth fall to less than 2% of daily requirements in the second year, remain between 1-2% of energy requirements until mid-adolescence, and become negligible by 20 years of age [Food and Agriculture Organization, 2001].

Figure 3 – Components of energy expenditure as percentage of metabolisable energy intake in each age group [Wells & Davies, 1998]

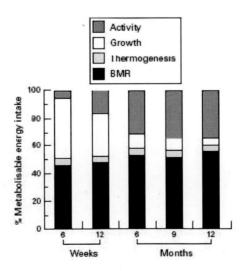

Reproduced from: Arch Dis Child, Wells JC & Davies PS, vol 78(2), pages 131-136, 1998, with permission from BMI Publishing Group Ltd.

103.	During lactation, as in pregnancy (section 3.1.2), the mother provides the nutritional needs of the growing infant. Adaptive changes including changes in absorption, metabolism and excretion of minerals, allow her to achieve this without a substantial increment in dietary intake.

104.	Growth is a dynamic process; a single measurement does not allow assessment. A series of measurements, including weight, height or length[xiii], and head circumference, must be plotted against time and interpreted by reference to population data (see section 3.5 *Influences on growth*).

105.	An increase in weight is often taken to indicate satisfactory progress of growth in a child, but variations in the composition of tissue deposited (i.e. muscle development and fat deposition) make interpretation of weight gain alone difficult. The usefulness of growth measurements also depends on accuracy of measurements. Readings of height and weight are subject to bias if the observer has preconceptions about the child's growth [Hall & Elliman, 2003].

3.3.1   Patterns of postnatal growth

106.	Figures 4 and 5 show schematically the growth profile of a typical child (length/height and weight) as described by Tanner. They indicate how the velocity of growth changes with age [Tanner, 1978] but are not intended to provide normative data. In reality, there is considerable variability within and between both girls and boys, particularly at puberty.

107.	Figure 4 shows that in early infancy, height velocity in boys is greater than in girls but becomes equal at about 7 months of age and subsequently lower at 4 years. From birth until age 4 to 5 years, the rate of growth in height declines rapidly, slightly faster in boys. The subsequent rise is related to puberty and there is considerable inter-individual variation in age at onset.

108.	The pattern of weight change is very similar. Figure 5 shows that boys' weight velocity is greater at birth, but becomes equal to girls' at about 8 months and then gradually drops below. Boys' weight then stays a little below girls' right up to adolescence. Weight velocity depends on more factors than height velocity, which makes generalisation to individual children difficult [Tanner *et al.*, 1966]. The peak velocity for the adolescent spurt in weight lags behind the peak velocity for height by about 3 months on average.

xiii For children up to 24 months of age, supine length is measured rather than standing height

Figure 4 – Velocity curves for supine length or height in boys or girls. These curves represent height growth velocity and how this changes with age, but are not intended to depict normative data [Tanner *et al.*, 1966]

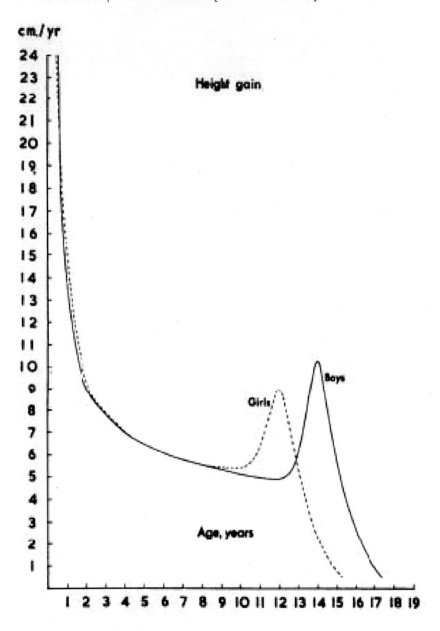

Reproduced from: Arch Dis Child, Tanner JM, Whitehouse RH & Takaishi M, vol 41, pages 454-471, 1966 with permission from BMJ Publishing Group Ltd.

Figure 5 – Velocity curves for weight in boys or girls. These curves represent the weight growth velocity and how this changes with age, but are not intended to depict normative data [Tanner et al., 1966]

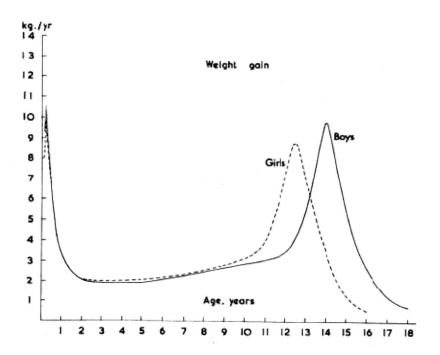

Reproduced from: Arch Dis Child, Tanner JM, Whitehouse RH & Takaishi M, vol 41, pages 454-471, 1966 with permission from BMJ Publishing Group Ltd.

109.   More recent velocity standards were produced by the World Health Organization (WHO) in 2009 (based on the same sample and statistical approaches as those used in the construction of the WHO attained growth standards published in 2006 – see section 3.5 *Influences on growth*). These provide standards for comparing the rapid and changing rate of growth in early childhood (0-2 years), regardless of ethnicity, socioeconomic status and type of feeding.

110.   Karlberg modelled the pattern of human growth from conception to completion as a set of three overlapping curves, termed the *infant, childhood* and *pubertal* phases [Karlberg, 1989]; this is known as the *infancy-childhood-puberty* (ICP) model of human growth (Figure 6 *The Karlberg ICP growth model for height for boys*).

111.   The three phases summate to form the combined growth curve, each phase commencing as the previous one attains peak velocity. The *infant* phase begins at conception and ends in early postnatal life; relative growth is more rapid during this phase than at any other time. The *childhood* phase begins after birth during the decelerating phase of the infant velocity curve and ends in adolescence. Finally, the *pubertal* phase begins with the onset of puberty and extends until growth and maturation are completed in adulthood.

Figure 6 – The Karlberg ICP growth model for height for boys. The mean functions are plotted for each of the three components as well as the combined growth. The average at onset of the childhood and puberty components were used. The interrupted curve at 3 years reflects the change in measuring position from lying to standing up (could have been given at 1 or 2 years, as well). The key hormones involved in the regulation of growth are also given [Karlberg *et al.*, 1994].

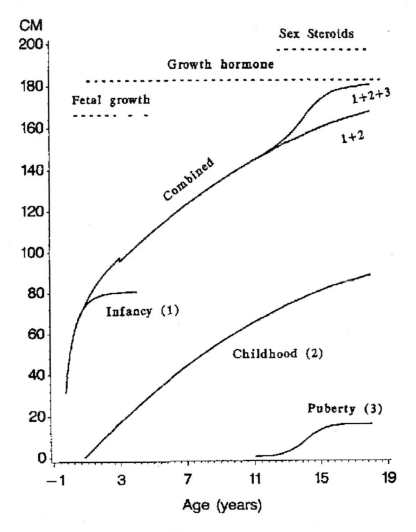

Reprinted by permission from Macmillan Publishers Ltd: Eur J Clin Nutr (Karlberg *et al.*, (1994) Linear growth retardation in relation to the three phases of growth. Eur J Clin Nutr, vol 48 Supp 1, pages S25-43. discussion S43-4), Copyright (1994).

112. The importance of distinguishing between these phases is that each relates to underlying genetic, hormonal and nutritional factors that influence growth, leading ultimately to differences in skeletal maturation and development in an individual child. Phases are additive and the age at onset is a critical factor in determining final adult height [Karlberg, 1989].

113. The greatest growth velocity occurs in the infant phase, which may be nutritionally led, and this accounts for the much greater vulnerability of young children to chronic energy and nutrient restriction. Restriction of growth at this stage results in stunting, which impacts negatively on adult height. Karlberg proposes that any delay in the transition from infant to childhood growth (see later section 3.4 *Growth faltering*) will also have profound effects on the attained height in subsequent years.

114. Organs and tissues do not grow at a uniform rate [Stratz, 1904]. A notable difference between an adult and an infant is the relative weight of the brain, which is growing at a peak velocity around term and completes most of its growth in the first two years of life. In the full-term newborn, it represents about 12% of the body weight, but in the adult is about 2%. In the presence of an adequate nutrient supply and the absence of ill health, these processes occur in a genetically predetermined and regulated sequence. Sexual differences in body composition become most marked after puberty but are present in earlier childhood too [Wells, 2000].

115. Although much individual variation occurs in the timing of the onset of puberty in both girls and boys, the overall sequence of pubertal events is well preserved [Tanner, 1953]. In girls, the pubertal growth spurt occurs between 8 and 13 years of age, soon after the initiation of breast development in the majority. In boys, the growth spurt occurs as a later pubertal phenomenon about one year after pubertal onset, defined by an increase in testicular volume [Tanner, 1953; Tanner *et al.*, 1976]. Therefore, growth may serve as a tool in the assessment of secular changes in pubertal timing, but must be considered separately for girls and boys. Moreover there is a need for careful assessment of pubertal staging when interpreting the growth pattern of individual children in adolescence.

116. It has been observed that girls with higher body weight, higher body mass index, more body fat, and greater height reach their menarche earlier [Koprowski *et al.*, 1999; Petridou *et al.*, 1996; Moisan *et al.*, 1990]. In the last two centuries, age at menarche has decreased in several European populations, whereas adult height has increased. Age at menarche in British adolescents has stabilised over the last 20-40 years or so [Whincup, 2001]. Those women who reach menarche relatively later eventually become taller adults, compared to those who undergo menarche earlier [Onland-Moret *et al.*, 2005]. A faster tempo of childhood growth, characterised by rapid weight gain and growth, leads to taller childhood stature and earlier menarche with consequent shorter adult stature. There may also be a transgenerational influence towards faster tempo of growth which is transmitted from the mother to the offspring [Ong *et al.*, 2007].

117. Early menarche is an established risk factor for breast cancer [World Cancer Research Fund / American Institute for Cancer Research, 2007]. The timing of menarche is also likely to be determined by a growth factor operating near the time of birth, which also affects later weight, but not height. The mechanisms involved in this are unclear [Cole, 2000].

3.4   Growth faltering

118.   In the fetus and young child, a period of energy and nutrient restriction or illness may impair growth. The faltering of growth *in utero* is termed *intrauterine growth restriction* (IUGR) and is detectable through serial ultrasonic measurement of fetal dimensions during the pregnancy. The term IUGR therefore describes velocity of growth and must be differentiated from attained size at birth. Infants who are born "small for gestational age" (SGA) (see section 3.2) may have been small throughout pregnancy yet grown at a normal velocity [Kramer, 2003]. Conversely some infants born at a weight appropriate for gestational age may have shown intrauterine growth restriction [Altman & Hytten, 1989; Kramer & Victora, 2001] (see section 3.2.3).

119.   Postnatal growth faltering is usually first evident as a fall in relative weight. This can be quantified as a change in standard deviation (SD) score or centile position over time and has been operationally defined in the UK as a fall in weight equating or exceeding 1.3 SD[xiv] during the first year of life. This change in relative centile position, or "centile crossing", is termed "conditional weight gain". The proportion of infants in any population who show centile crossing, is dependent firstly on the growth reference chosen and, secondly, on weight at birth. As a group, infants who are heavier at birth are more likely to show downward centile crossing; and those who are lighter at birth are more likely to show upward centile crossing [Wright *et al*., 1994; Cole, 1995; Scientific Advisory Committee on Nutrition, 2007a].

3.4.1   Canalisation, catch-up and catch-down growth

120.   In the context of human growth, the term *"canalisation"* describes the tendency to follow a genetically determined trajectory, given optimal health conditions and nutrient supply. Individuals whose growth has slowed or accelerated as a consequence of disease or other influences, show a tendency to accelerate or decelerate once these influences are removed [Prader *et al*., 1963]. Rapid growth following a period of restriction is termed *catch-up growth* and may ultimately redress wholly or partly the accrued deficit in weight and size.

121.   The term "catch-up" is also used to describe the relatively rapid early postnatal growth observed in infants who have been subjected to intrauterine growth restriction. In contrast, "catch-down", a relatively slow rate of postnatal growth, may be observed in infants who have shown intrauterine growth acceleration leading to macrosomia (for example the infant of a diabetic mother). Whilst "catch-up" from low birthweight may be beneficial in the short term to child survival [Pelletier *et al*., 1993] it has been speculated that such *compensatory* growth may impose physiological costs on the organism by programming [Lucas *et al*., 1999; Victora & Barros, 2001]. The associated disease costs may not be evident until later in life [Metcalfe & Monaghan, 2001].

122.   Catch-up and catch-down growth have both biological and statistical components. Statistically, the phenomenon of regression to the mean predicts that children

---

xiv This distance is equivalent to two "centile spaces" on the "nine-centile" chart which is formatted such that each centile line is positioned at a fixed distance of 0.66SD from the line above or below [Cole, 1994].

initially at the extremes of the distribution converge towards the mean over time. The chance of this happening can be predicted from the population reference distribution, allowing the quantification of a separate biological component over and above that expected statistically [Cameron *et al.*, 2005]. Catch-up growth after intrauterine constraint or restriction is usually completed by the end of the first year of life, but in extreme cases may continue into the second year.

123.   Catch-up and catch-down growth are common phenomena during infancy [Wright *et al.*, 1994; Cole, 1995]. A retrospective analysis of 10,844 US children born in the 1960s and 70s showed that 39% of children crossed two major percentiles[xv] for weight-for-age in their first 6 months, and 32% crossed two major percentiles for height-for-age in the first 6 months. Such percentile crossing was less common from 6 to 24 months of age, and least common among those 24 to 60 months of age [Mei *et al.*, 2004].

124.   It is important to consider the catch-up process not only in terms of weight or height, but also in terms of the type of tissue deposited. Postnatal catch-up growth may lead to differences in body composition relative to infants not exhibiting catch-up growth. For example, several prospective studies have observed the progressive deposition of more abdominal fat and increasing body adiposity in later childhood and adulthood after a period of catch-up growth during infancy [Ong *et al.*, 2000; Reilly *et al.*, 2005; Ibanez *et al.*, 2006; Karaolis-Danckert *et al.*, 2006; McCarthy *et al.*, 2007].

125.   Tanner described two ways in which an individual might demonstrate complete catch-up following pre or postnatal growth restriction. Growth may be accelerated (as above); or bone maturation and bone growth delayed, sometimes in association with a delay in the onset of puberty [Tanner, 1981]. Frequently, catch-up is a mixture of these short-term and long-term processes. The extent to which they are distinct, and the mechanisms which underlie them, remain unclear.

126.   Catch-up growth may be complete or incomplete, depending on both the timing and duration of the constraining stimulus and the extent to which conditions are optimised during recovery. Generally the earlier nutritional restriction occurs, and the more prolonged its duration, the less likely complete catch-up will occur. This is to a large extent a corollary of the shape of the growth velocity curve: a greater deficit is more quickly accrued during a period normally characterised by rapid growth. Equally, growth must accelerate by a relatively greater amount to restore the deficit once the child is older, because normal velocity will have slowed (see section 3.3.1 *Patterns of postnatal growth*).

3.4.2   Critical periods and programming in humans

127.   Tissues and organs in the fetal body appear to undergo "critical" [Widdowson & McCance, 1975] or "sensitive" periods [Tanner, 1990] of development, where insults or stimuli at a given time lead to lifelong changes in organ structure or function [Lucas, 1991]. In the physiological sense, they represent stages of life at which

---

xv   The 5th, 10th, 25th, 50th, 75th, 90th and 95th percentiles were defined as the major percentiles in this study.

there is increased sensitivity of a receptor to a highly specific stimulus, followed by decreasing sensitivity and eventually by no response. For example, in the 14th postmenstrual week, the human male fetus must receive male sex hormones to stimulate the differentiation of the external reproductive organs.

128. The critical period hypothesis posits that, once past, a developmental opportunity is lost and phenotypic attributes are set. Historically, human critical growth periods occurring *in utero* were considered to have more long-term implications than those occurring postnatally, although this may have reflected lesser ability to detect the latter [Tanner, 1990]. It has been stated that *"programming is the consequence of the innate capacity of developing tissues to adapt to the conditions that prevail during early life, which for almost all cell types in all organs is an ability that is present for only a short period before the time of birth"* [Langley-Evans, 2006]

129. Critical periods may originate with periods of rapid cell division when a change in fetal substrate supply could be expected to exert maximal effect on growth and differentiation. Nutritional programming can thus be considered a subtle and complex metabolic response by the fetus to nutrient-gene interactions during such a period of *developmental plasticity*. The organism's ability to change its phenotype in response to changes in the environment explains how a range of physiological or morphological phenotypes may arise from a single genotype as the consequence of exposure to different environmental conditions [Horton, 2005].

130. Experimental and observational research in humans and other species demonstrates the importance of early development for later health outcomes [Lucas, 1994; Lucas, 1998; Godfrey & Barker, 2000] (see also Chapters 4 and 5). Empirical studies in animals have shown that different organs have different critical periods of development. Thus insults or stimuli delivered at a specific time, lead to reproducible lifelong changes in organ structure or function [Lucas, 1991].

131. Key evidence about the vulnerability of humans stems from observations on the offspring of mothers who experienced wartime famine at known points in gestation. The Dutch hunger winter of 1944 resulted in severe food shortage for a period of 5-6 months, whereas the siege of Leningrad was much more prolonged lasting some 2 years between 1941 and 1944.

132. Studies of pregnancies occurring during the Dutch famine of 1944-1945 found that the offspring effects of maternal food shortage varied with the period of gestation at which it occurred [Lumey et al., 1993]. Mothers with severely restricted energy and nutrient intakes (Dutch hunger winter, 1944-45) during late gestation tended to bear offspring with lower birthweight and size (crown-heel length and head circumference) [Stein et al., 2004]. Birth size and body proportions were not affected by first trimester famine exposure.

133.   Famine exposure during early gestation was associated with decreased factor VII[xvi] plasma concentrations [Roseboom *et al.*, 2000c], increased serum cholesterol concentrations and coronary heart disease (CHD) risk [Roseboom *et al.*, 2000b; Roseboom *et al.*, 2000a] in later adult life. Exposure in mid-gestation was associated with renal dysfunction (microalbuminuria) [Painter *et al.*, 2005] and prevalence of obstructive airways disease [Lopuhaa *et al.*, 2000]. Late gestational exposure was associated with decreased glucose tolerance in adulthood, especially among those who became obese in later life [Ravelli *et al.*, 1998]. No association was observed between prenatal famine exposure at any stage of gestation and blood pressure in adulthood [Roseboom *et al.*, 1999].

134.   These findings suggest that the timing of prenatal exposure to famine determines which organ system is affected. The health outcome may reflect which critical periods of rapid growth and development coincided with the famine exposure. For example, there is normally a rapid increase in nephron number in mid-gestation and famine exposure at this point was associated with renal dysfunction in later life [Painter *et al.*, 2005].

135.   Offspring fingerprints may be morphological markers of altered intrauterine growth processes relevant to the early prenatal origins of several chronic diseases [Godfrey *et al.*, 1993; Kahn *et al.*, 2008]. A report from the Dutch Hunger Winter Families Study found that diabetes in adults over 55 years of age was associated with a fingerprint characteristic known to be established in early pregnancy, irrespective of birthweight [Kahn *et al.*, 2009]. The association was conserved even amongst those diagnosed in the preceding 7 years.

136.   Initial results from the Dutch famine studies suggested intergenerational associations: it was reported that mothers exposed to famine as first and second trimester fetuses had offspring with birthweights lower than mothers who had not been exposed to famine *in utero* [Lumey, 1992] (see also section 3.1.1 *Determinants of fetal growth*). A subsequent study failed to confirm such an association [Stein & Lumey, 2000].

137.   Intrauterine and early infant (from 10 weeks of age) exposure to food shortage during the siege of Leningrad (1941-4) was not associated with glucose intolerance, dyslipidaemia, hypertension nor cardiovascular disease in adult life [Stanner *et al.*, 1997; Stanner & Yudkin, 2001]. The authors attributed this to a lack of early childhood catch-up growth after the Leningrad famine, in contrast to the situation that prevailed in Holland.

138.   Overall, these extreme conditions seem of greater contemporary relevance to populations in developing countries than industrialised nations. The majority of low birthweight babies are born in developing countries [de Onis *et al.*, 1998], though the example of Japan (see section 3.2.2) illustrates that important exceptions may occur. Behavioural eating disorders e.g. bulimia nervosa, during pregnancy have

---

xvi Factor VII is one of the vitamin K-dependent coagulation factors synthesized principally in the liver and secreted as a single-chain glycoprotein.

also been associated with low birthweight and intrauterine growth restriction [Conti *et al.*, 1998; James, 2001].

3.5   Influences on growth

139.   Growth monitoring is pivotal to fetal and child health surveillance. A healthy, well-nourished child can be expected to follow a trajectory, which parallels the genetically determined centile.

140.   The distinction between attained weight or size and growth is crucial. Measurements of current weight and size show where an individual is in relation to a population distribution, but do not describe the rate of growth. Growth velocity cannot be estimated from fewer than two accurate measurements spaced sufficiently far apart in time.

141.   Growth charts are used to document the growth of infants, children and adolescents. They are usually formatted as a series of percentile curves (for weight, height and head circumference) that illustrate the population distribution of selected body measurements.

142.   The UK1990 growth reference was based on cross-sectional measurements of several thousand British children in seven studies performed between 1972 and 1989. The charts depicted measurements of weight, height, BMI, head circumference and stages of puberty, between birth and twenty years [Cole *et al.*, 1998].

143.   It has been widely acknowledged that the growth pattern of exclusively breastfed infants varied from that depicted by former UK and US growth charts [Whitehead & Paul, 1984; Dewey *et al.*, 1995]. It is now recognised that the UK and US charts were based on a high proportion of infants in the UK and USA who were formula or mixed-fed at the time the reference data were collected. On the UK1990 and National Health Center for Health Statistics (US) growth charts, breastfed babies appeared to cross centiles upwards in the early months, and cross downwards through centiles in the second half of infancy [Hediger *et al.*, 2000; Cole *et al.*, 2002]. In consequence, breastfed babies appeared lighter on these charts at 12 months by as much as half a centile space as a group compared to formula-fed infants [Scientific Advisory Committee on Nutrition, 2007a].

144.   In 2007, the Department of Health accepted recommendations from the Joint SACN/Royal College of Paediatrics and Child Health (RCPCH) Expert Group to replace the UK1990 reference with the new World Health Organisation (WHO) Growth Standards [Scientific Advisory Committee on Nutrition, 2007a]. These reflect the growth of healthy term infants from six countries who were exclusively or predominantly breastfed for the first 4-6 months of life (mean age at the start of complementary feeding 5.4 months). The new charts were introduced to the UK in May 2009 because they represent an international *standard* of growth for all healthy infants and young children however they are fed. These charts are in current use to monitor all UK children up the age of 4 years.

145. The difference between a reference and a standard is fundamental. A growth *reference* simply describes the growth pattern of a sample of children in the general population regardless of health or social status, whereas a growth *standard* describes the growth of a 'healthy' population and suggests an aspirational model or target. In the first half of infancy, the pattern of growth shown by infants exclusively breastfed represents a biological norm being associated globally with short-, medium- and long-term health outcomes superior to those of infants artificially fed [Scientific Advisory Committee on Nutrition, 2007a].

3.5.1 Secular trends in growth

146. During the 20th century, secular increases in height have been observed among children and adults in the UK. Increments of 10-30 mm have been observed with each succeeding decade [Chinn & Rona, 1984; Kuh *et al.*, 1991; Cole, 2000]. Adult height is linked to genetic factors, birthweight, rate of growth, age at puberty and environmental factors, such as diet. There has also been a concomitant change in weight, both in adults and in children. Secular changes in height have slowed in Northern Europe, while weight continues to increase as indicated by the population trend towards increasing BMI [Cole, 2003].

147. In some European countries, the secular trend to greater height has stopped. One explanation is that the genetic height potential of the population has been reached. It has been suggested that this approximates a population mean of 1.8 metres in northern European countries [Larnkjaer, *et al.*, 2006]. An analysis of conscript height in European countries found that a secular increase in height stopped approximately 18 years after neonatal mortality had fallen below 4/1000 deliveries [Schmidt *et al.*, 1995].

148. Appendicular growth predominates during pre-pubertal years, including infancy, and axial growth during puberty [Tanner, 1990]. The cessation of limb growth and acceleration of truncal growth at puberty are sex-hormone dependent due to effects on the action of growth hormone and IGF.

149. Intergenerational increases in height are generally due to increased leg length, which is linked to growth during infancy [Gunnell *et al.*, 2001]. Leg growth is mediated by the expression of growth-hormone receptors on the growth plates during infancy, and this may be affected by the interaction between concurrent nutrition and the nominal growth rate set during pregnancy. Thus leg length in adult life tends to reflect the operation of early life factors; in the 1946 British birth cohort it was positively associated with breastfeeding and energy intake at the age of 4 years [Wadsworth *et al.*, 2002]. During puberty, truncal growth becomes more prominent [Tanner, 1990].

150. Nutritional factors could thus influence disease risk by affecting the endocrine regulation of growth, for example by modulating IGF-1 secretion. Adult height would thus act as a marker of early life experience [Marmot *et al.*, 1984]. Undernutrition in early life is also associated with a delay in the transition from infant to childhood growth and consequent reduction of attained height [Karlberg, 1989] (see earlier section 3.3.1 *Patterns of postnatal growth*).

3.5.2 Effects of early feeding on growth

151. Observational studies have described associations between method of infant feeding and growth pattern in early life, particularly during infancy.

152. A large (17,046 term mother-baby pairs) controlled trial in Belarus allocated hospitals to participate or not in the WHO/Unicef Baby Friendly Initiative. The intervention significantly increased the proportion of infants breastfed exclusively or predominantly for more than 3 months [Kramer *et al.*, 2001]. Observational data were later collected on a cohort of infants nested within this trial. These showed that infants fed infant formula or other milk showed faster gain in weight and length throughout infancy. A dose-response gradient was observed, and the strongest associations were apparent at 3 to 6 months [Kramer *et al.*, 2004]. Reverse causality (for example cessation of breastfeeding in hungrier babies) or the operation of confounding factors could not be excluded as the data were observational.

153. A subsequent comparison was based on 13,889 infants followed up at age 6.5 years of age [Kramer *et al.*, 2007]. This revealed no differences in physical parameters (weight, height, BMI, waist and hip circumferences, skinfolds) or blood pressure between babies born in intervention or control hospitals, despite the greater prevalence of exclusive breastfeeding in the former group (see section 5.1 *Human intervention studies*). It was suggested that associations reported in earlier analyses and other observational studies may be the result of confounding and selection bias.

154. Several studies have shown that serum IGF-1 concentrations are lower in breastfed compared with formula-fed infants [Chellakooty *et al.*, 2006], at 3 months, 4 to 8 months [Savino *et al.*, 2005], and at 6 months of age [Socha *et al.*, 2005]. Formula has a higher protein content than breastmilk [Heinig *et al.*, 1993] and it is plausible that this stimulates IGF-1 secretion and infant growth [Axelsson *et al.*, 1989; Hoppe *et al.*, 2006]. A lower infant IGF-1 concentration is consistent with the observation that breastfed infants gain weight more slowly than formula-fed infants in late infancy. However, some data indicate that adults who were breastfed as infants tend to be taller [Martin *et al.*, 2002; Victora *et al.*, 2003].

155. Higher protein intake during infancy has been associated with rapid early weight gain and later obesity [Koletzko *et al.*, 2005] though results from the Southampton Women's Survey, which measured body fat using dual energy x-ray absorptiometry (DXA), has suggested that protein intake in infancy is not associated with adiposity in later childhood at 4 years [Robinson *et al.*, 2008].

156. Findings from the Avon Longitudinal Study of Parents and Children (ALSPAC) cohort in the UK showed a significant association between serum IGF-1 concentrations measured at 7 to 8 years of life and the history of breastfeeding. Compared with those who had never been breastfed, children who had been partially breastfed or exclusively breastfed for at least 2 months, had significantly *higher* IGF-1 concentrations [Martin *et al.*, 2005c; Schack-Nielsen & Michaelsen, 2007]. Serum IGF-1 was also strongly positively associated with growth in height from 5 years to

9-10 years of age [Rogers *et al.*, 2006]. It was suggested that breastfeeding might programme the IGF axis.

157. The effects of complementary feeding and early introduction of solid foods (usually associated with early formula feeding) on growth remain unclear [Hamlyn *et al.*, 2002; Foster *et al.*, 1997]. Observational data collected from over 1600 infants recruited to five UK prospective randomised trials of formula feeding were used to examine the relationships between age at introduction of solid foods, growth and health outcomes up to 18 months. Infants introduced to solid foods earlier were larger at 12 weeks than those introduced later, but the growth trajectories of the two groups 'converged' at 18 months [Morgan *et al.*, 2004].

158. A limited number of RCTs have explored the effect of infant feeding on growth in infancy. Some have additionally examined cardiovascular risk factors in later childhood but not in adult life. These studies are summarised in section 5.1.

3.6   Summary

159. The pattern of growth and development between conception and achievement of adulthood, reflects interaction between genetic and environmental influences, including nutrient supply, on human growth and development.

160. The high velocity of growth and development during fetal and early postnatal life (before the age of about 2 years) implies that restriction of nutrient supply will have greatest effect at these stages of life.

161. Development occurs in an ordered sequence, so that the separate organs and tissues of the body achieve maximal growth velocity at different stages of development. Organs and tissues are most vulnerable to nutrient restriction at these points which have been termed "critical periods" of development.

162. Nutrient restriction during development can result in irreversible alteration of organ and tissue architecture and function. The consequence of such changes is "programming" of an individual's phenotype, evident as alteration of body structure, composition and metabolic competence.

163. Many determinants of fetal growth are established prior to pregnancy, during the immediate periconceptional period or the earlier life course of the mother. A woman's nutritional status at the commencement of pregnancy will determine her ability to meet the needs of the fetus from dietary intake and tissue nutrient reserves.

164. During pregnancy, many major physiological and metabolic changes occur in the mother. These work together to conserve fetal nutrient supply. They include adaptations which increase uptake of nutrients from the diet, reduce excretion and alter maternal nutrient partitioning in favour of the fetoplacental unit.

165. Despite these adaptations, maternal nutrient restriction may impact on weight, size, body composition and later health of the offspring, particularly when it is severe, for example as in famine or anorexia. Low maternal status for some

micronutrients has some characterised effects on human pregnancy (for example in the case of vitamin D and folate) but the specific effects of deficiency in many other individual nutrients are currently not well understood.

166. Pathological and environmental factors (such as smoking and altitude) may impair placental function and restrict the growth of the fetus even in the presence of adequate maternal dietary supply.

167. Birthweight is frequently used as a measure of fetal outcome but has many limitations as a descriptor of offspring phenotype. Low birthweight (defined by a birthweight of less than 2500g) may be attributable to shortening of gestation (premature birth) or to slowing of fetal growth (intrauterine growth restriction; IUGR).

168. Intrauterine growth restriction is not necessarily marked by low birthweight. For example, a fetus which is large in early pregnancy may grow relatively slowly and yet attain a birthweight within the normal range of the population in question.

169. Infants who showed restriction of growth *in utero* frequently differ in body composition from those who did not. These differences may be evident in body dimensions (such as length and head circumference) and the relative amounts or distribution of tissues within the body.

170. Postnatal catch-up (or "compensatory") growth following intrauterine restriction, may amplify differences in body composition. This potentially has additional implications for metabolic function and disease risk.

171. The type of feeding in infancy also influences both the rate of growth and the type of tissue deposited. Early nutrient exposure may thus induce effects on body composition or hormonal axes and regulate the pattern of childhood growth. The extent to which genetic and ethnic variation influences these processes is currently not clear.

4 Impact of early nutrition on later chronic disease outcomes: epidemiological studies

172. The following sections examine the epidemiological evidence relating to the impact of early nutrition on a range of chronic disease outcomes. Birthweight, placental weight and measures of size or body composition at birth have all been related to disease outcomes and risk factors for chronic disease in adult life. The impact of various other pre- and postnatal factors, including maternal nutrient intake, early postnatal growth and feeding, are also considered.

173. The largest body of epidemiological evidence is associated with cardiovascular disease outcomes such as coronary heart disease and stroke, cancer and type 2 diabetes. These form the primary focus of the following sections. When evaluating the evidence, the consistency and strength of associations is considered and limitations highlighted.

4.1 Contribution of the epidemiological evidence

174. Epidemiological studies can only demonstrate that a factor is associated with the incidence of disease in the exposed population. They have limited potential for causal inference, but can help frame research questions to help establish causality. The findings of epidemiological studies cannot always be generalised beyond the population studied.

175. It is not always clear whether intermediate outcomes or biological markers, which are often used as proxy measures in epidemiology, are truly predictive of the health outcome that they are considered to indicate. For example, there is a varying degree of correlation between BMI at different stages of childhood and adult BMI (see section 2.1.1). Despite this, epidemiology can usefully suggest further avenues of research.

4.1.1 Methodological issues in observational studies (see also Chapter 2 Methodological Considerations)

176. Birthweight is commonly used in epidemiological studies with the implication that it represents a summary measure of fetal nutritional exposure. However, birthweight is neither a sensitive nor a specific measure of fetal nutrient supply. Birthweight may vary for many reasons (see section 3.2 *Birthweight*). Moreover, animal studies have shown that variation of maternal dietary intake may alter the offspring's nutritional phenotype without modification of birthweight.

177. The large sample sizes that are characteristic of epidemiological research generally necessitate the use of anthropometric measurements as indicators of body composition. The limitations of anthropometric ratios (such as body mass index,

BMI, or ponderal index, PI) as indicators of fat mass or fat-free mass need to be emphasised. Central adiposity is considered a stronger indicator of cardiovascular risk [Daniels et al., 1999; Wells et al., 2007b] but BMI provides no information about body shape, pattern of fat distribution or fat to lean mass ratio.

178. Although BMI is often used as a measure of adiposity in children, cautious interpretation is required when comparing groups that differ in age or when predicting an individual's fat mass [Pietrobelli et al., 1998]. Children of the same age and gender can have a two-fold range of fat mass for a given BMI value whether obese or not [Wells et al., 2007a].

179. Many individual studies (both observational and experimental) have limited statistical power to detect modest associations. Imprecise measures of primary exposure may also obscure true associations with disease outcomes.

180. Conversely there is some evidence of publication bias leading to inappropriate emphasis on studies yielding extreme results [Huxley et al., 2002]. Publication bias has been asserted in reporting of the relationships between blood pressure and birthweight [Huxley et al., 2002], and infant feeding pattern [Owen et al., 2003a]. This problem may have been compounded by the failure of published studies to present quantitative data on associations considered unimpressive [Huxley et al., 2002]. This tendency of null studies to avoid stating regression coefficients may introduce bias in meta-analysis.

181. The scientific literature about impact of early feeding uses definitions, which are often inconsistent, particularly in relation to breastfeeding. For example, 'breastfeeding' may indicate either exclusive breastfeeding[xvii] or breastfeeding alongside the use of infant formula (mixed feeding[xviii]) and other foods and fluids. Likewise the term 'weaning' can be used either in its contemporary sense to denote the introduction of foods other than breastmilk or infant formula [Department of Health, 1994] or its more historical sense describing weaning from the breast. 'Complementary feeding'[xix] is now preferred as a term to denote infant dietary diversification but is less commonly used. Additionally retrospective rather than prospective recording of infant feeding practices may introduce bias.

182. In studies with many early exposure measurements (particularly those with detailed birth and childhood records), multiple hypothesis testing increases the possibility of false positive associations [Paneth & Susser, 1995]. Many studies lack adjustment for confounding factors; social circumstances at different stages of the lifecourse are particularly important potential confounders [Huxley et al., 2002]. Limited response and follow-up rates may also give rise to ascertainment or sampling bias [Joseph & Kramer, 1996; Susser & Levin, 1999].

xvii Exclusive breastfeeding is when an infant receives only breastmilk and may be given drops or syrups consisting of vitamins, mineral supplements or medicines but no other food or liquids. UK Health Departments recommend exclusive breastfeeding for the first six months of an infant's life [Department of Health, 2003].

xviii Mixed feeding refers to when an infant receives both breastmilk and infant formula milk.

xix Complementary feeding refers to the process of diversifying diet by introduction of foods other than milk.

183. Inadequate adjustment for confounders, e.g. socioeconomic status, may lead to spurious associations being made. Confounding by social factors associated with breastfeeding is one example [Wells *et al.*, 2007a]: some observational studies reporting slower growth in breastfed infants relative to formula-fed infants have not adjusted adequately for confounding factors such as socioeconomic influences, maternal smoking in pregnancy, and maternal BMI [Kramer *et al.*, 2002].

184. Alternatively, inappropriate adjustment for exposures on the causal pathway, e.g. weight or height, may lead to estimates that amplify effect sizes. Current weight is associated with both the outcome variable (cardiovascular risk) and the predictor variable (birthweight). There may be further confounding, where, for example, associations weaken with age [Whincup, 1998; Huxley *et al.*, 2002; Tu *et al.*, 2005].

185. Some of these concerns have been refuted in specific studies. For example, the relation between birthweight and CHD has been observed in a Finnish study with a high follow-up rate without adjustment for current body weight or size [Eriksson *et al.*, 2001]; data from a Swedish cohort suggests that the relationship between birthweight and CHD is not confounded by adult social class [Leon *et al.*, 1998].

186. Limitations in measuring exposure, coupled with the methodological problems intrinsic to human life-course epidemiology make it difficult to ascribe mechanisms to any associations observed, but raise important hypotheses, which can be tested empirically in controlled human and animal studies.

187. A more general problem is the lack of clear agreement between observational studies on: (i) the overall strength and importance of different maternal, fetal and child exposures in the aetiology of disease risk, and (ii) the intermediate components of the disease risk pathway, which are mediating the effects of early life factors. Understanding the latter requires a clear understanding of the biological mechanisms that link exposure to outcome.

4.2   Cardiovascular disease (CVD)

188. Cohort studies in the UK have observed an inverse association between infant weight, within the normal range, and adult cardiovascular disease (CVD) risk in males [Barker *et al.*, 1989a; Barker *et al.*, 1989b; Hales & Ozanne, 2003]. The association between lower birthweight and increased CVD risk was later replicated in other cohorts and in other countries. It was later shown that adjustment for length of gestation increased the strength of association with CVD risk in adulthood, suggesting that fetal growth rate was more important than gestational length in determining future CVD risk [Eriksson *et al.*, 1999; Forsen *et al.*, 1999].

4.2.1   Coronary heart disease (CHD)

4.2.1.1   Birthweight, size and body composition at birth and CHD

189. A systematic review and meta-analysis of observational studies (18 studies all from developed countries apart from one in India, total of 147,009 people) observed an inverse association between birthweight and subsequent development of ischaemic heart disease (IHD) (outcomes included IHD, CHD and CVD) in adulthood.

Overall age- and sex-adjusted relative risk (RR) of IHD was 0.84 (95% CI 0.81, 0.88) per 1kg increment in birthweight (p<0.0001) [Huxley et al., 2007] (Figure 7). This did not differ between men and women, and adjustment for potential confounders (including social class) did not alter the strength of association.

Figure 7 – Relative risks and 95% CIs for risk of ischemic heart disease (IHD) associated with 1 kg higher birthweight. First author [and reference] are as cited in the original Huxley et al., 2007 paper. The individual study estimates are of the association between birthweight and IHD incidence (fatal and nonfatal combined) or, when not available, IHD mortality or prevalence. The statistical size of the study was defined in terms of the inverse of the variance of the regression coefficient. Black squares indicate the point estimate for each study (with area proportional to statistical size), and the horizontal lines indicate the 95% CI for the observed effect. The dotted vertical line is the inverse variance–weighted regression through the overall point estimate, which is denoted as a diamond, representing the 95% CI [Huxley et al., 2007].

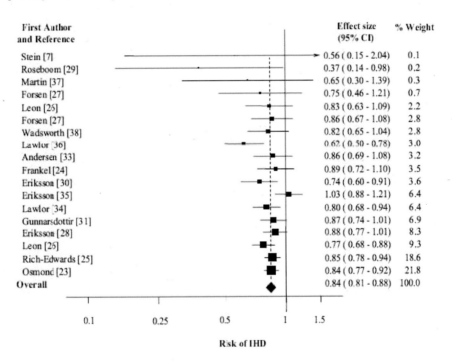

190. One cohort study, not included in this review, also reported a strong inverse association between birthweight and CHD (p=0.0005), but only among those above the highest tertile of BMI in later life [Frankel et al., 1996b]. Another cohort study reported a statistically insignificant association [Fall et al., 1995],

191. The Nurse's Health Cohort Study (included in the Huxley review) found that a higher BMI in adulthood was more strongly associated with risk for CHD among

women who were small at birth than those who were not [Rich-Edwards *et al.*, 2005].

192. Some studies have shown that other measures of size and body composition at birth show stronger associations with adult cardiovascular outcome and risk. For example, low ponderal index at birth increases the risk of some cardiovascular outcomes, particularly CHD [Forsen *et al.*, 1997] and a decreased abdominal circumference at birth has been associated positively with raised serum triacylglycerol concentrations at 50 years of age [Barker *et al.*, 1993].

4.2.1.2   Postnatal growth or size and CHD

193. A systematic review and meta-analysis of published studies from developed countries related BMI between age 2-30 years to later CHD risk (15 studies involving 731,337 participants and 23,894 CHD events). It revealed a non-statistically significant inverse association between BMI in early childhood (2-6 years) and later CHD risk (RR 0.94, 95% CI 0.82, 1.07) [Owen *et al.*, 2009b]. However, a consistently positive relationship was found from 7 years of age: BMI in later childhood (7 to <18 years) and in early adult life (18-30 years) were both positively related to later CHD risk (RR 1.09, 95% CI 1.00, 1.20; RR 1.19, 95% CI 1.11, 1.29 respectively) (Figure 8). These associations were not affected by adjustment for cigarette smoking, social class, blood pressure or blood cholesterol, and there was little effect of gender and year of birth. The authors reported considerable heterogeneity between study estimates.

Figure 8 – Relative risk (95% CI) of coronary outcome for a 1 kg/m² increase in BMI (including studies with repeat measures of BMI). Box area of each study is proportional to the inverse of the variance, with horizontal lines showing the 95% CI. First author (and reference number) as cited in the original Owen *et al.*, 2009b paper is indicated on the y-axis, for males (M), females (F), mean age in ascending order of BMI assessment (years) [Owen *et al.*, 2009b]

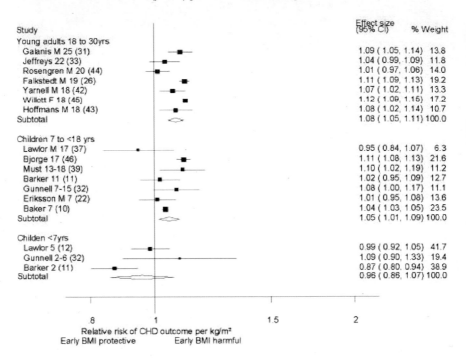

194. Another systematic review, identifying four cohort studies (2 UK, 2 Finnish) relating infant size or growth to IHD found that larger weight, height and BMI at 1 year were associated with reduced rates of ischaemic heart disease (IHD) in men but not in women [Fisher *et al.*, 2006]. This association was independent of weight at birth.

195. One of the studies included in this review described a Finnish cohort in which weight and height were measured in the first year and nine more times until 12 years of age [Eriksson *et al.*, 2001]. Boys who developed CHD in adulthood tended to be smaller than average at birth and remained so in infancy, but showed accelerated gain in weight and body mass index (BMI) thereafter. A broadly similar growth pattern was observed among girls in the same cohort who later developed CHD. The risk of CHD events in adulthood was thus related more to the tempo of change in BMI during childhood than the BMI at any particular age [Barker *et al.*, 2005].

196. A long-term follow-up study also identified associations between BMI in adolescence and later CHD risk [Engeland *et al.*, 2003]. This may however be

explained by the strong correlation of adolescent and adult body mass index [Guo & Chumlea, 1999].

197. Body mass index in childhood is consistently related longitudinally to markers of CHD risk in young adults including increased total and low density lipoprotein (LDL) cholesterol concentrations, blood pressure, insulin resistance, levels of haemostatic factors and lower high density lipoprotein (HDL) cholesterol concentration [Srinivasan et al., 1996; Berenson et al., 1998]. Cardiovascular risk profiles may be especially unfavourable in children with central adiposity [Daniels et al., 1999].

198. Taller adults have lower all-cause mortality rates [Waaler, 1984; Floud et al., 1990; Jousilahti et al., 2000] and a reduced CVD risk relative to shorter people [Paffenbarger & Wing, 1969; Wannamethee et al., 1998; Forsen et al., 2000; Jousilahti et al., 2000; Goldbourt & Tanne, 2002; McCarron et al., 2002]. Observed associations between height and CVD risk tend to point in the opposite direction to those observed with cancer (see section 4.5).

199. Studies from the UK Boyd Orr cohort suggest that leg length may be the component of stature generating these associations. Increases in childhood leg length, but not trunk length, were associated with decreased coronary heart disease mortality, but increased cancer risk in later life [Gunnell et al., 1998a; Gunnell et al., 1998b]. This suggests an effect of factors affecting the rate of growth in infancy and early childhood (see section 3.5.1).

4.2.1.3   Early feeding and CHD

200. A meta-analysis of observational (cohort) studies from developed countries, combined with results from the UK Boyd Orr Cohort, showed little evidence of an association of breastfeeding with later all-cause mortality (pooled ratio 1.01, 95% CI 0.91, 1.13) or cardiovascular mortality (1.96, 95% CI 0.94, 1.20) [Martin et al., 2004a]. Currently there is inconsistent evidence that being breastfed influences adult cardiovascular mortality.

201. It is difficult to establish the independent influence of early introduction of solid foods on cardiovascular risk and cardiovascular outcome in later life, as formula-fed infants tend to be introduced to solids earlier those breastfed [Foster et al., 1997; Hamlyn et al., 2002]; the influence of diet quality at this stage is also unclear.

202. Observational studies of men and women born in Hertfordshire in the early part of the 20th century, have shown that men who were "weaned"[xx] from breastmilk beyond one year had lower rates of CHD in adult life, compared to those "weaned" earlier [Fall, 1992; Osmond et al., 1993]. These findings have not been replicated [Wingard et al., 1994].

[xx]   "Weaning" is not explicitly defined in the paper. It generally defines the act of substituting other food for the milk, but may also imply cessation of breastfeeding.

4.2.1.4   Social factors and CHD

203. Several studies have reported that adverse social circumstances in childhood or adulthood are related to both prevalence [Wannamethee *et al.*, 1996] and incidence of CHD [Smith *et al.*, 1990; Hebert *et al.*, 1993; Wannamethee *et al.*, 1996; Brunner *et al.*, 1999]. Nevertheless the associations between postnatal growth rate and CVD (see section 4.2.1.2) persist in a number of studies after adjustment for markers of social status, including occupation [Fall *et al.*, 1995; Stein *et al.*, 1996; Frankel *et al.*, 1996b; Frankel *et al.*, 1996a; Leon *et al.*, 1998; Koupilova *et al.*, 1999].

4.2.2   Blood pressure

4.2.2.1   Maternal nutrient intake and blood pressure

204. A review identified five studies examining the relationship between maternal calcium intake and offspring blood pressure. Meta-analysis was conducted on four that provided data (2 observational studies and 2 RCTs). This showed a weak association between higher maternal calcium intake in pregnancy and lower offspring blood pressure, although the pooled estimate of mean difference was not statistically significant (−0.83 mmHg, 95% CI − 2.06, 4.0) [Brion *et al.*, 2008a].

205. A further review of maternal calcium supplementation trials conducted in the USA, Argentina, Australia and Gambia similarly identified little evidence of any effect of maternal calcium supplementation on offspring blood pressure [Hawkesworth, 2009].

206. In the Project Viva cohort study conducted in Massachusetts, United States, there was an inverse association between second-trimester supplemental maternal calcium intake and systolic blood pressure in offspring at 6 months. At 6 months of age, a systolic blood pressure difference of −3.0 mmHg (95% CI −4.9, −1.1) was observed for each 500 mg increment in maternal calcium intake during pregnancy. However, by 3 years of age no association between maternal calcium intake during pregnancy and offspring blood pressure was apparent [Bakker *et al.*, 2008].

207. The Brion *et al.* (2008a) review also identified five studies of maternal prenatal protein and carbohydrate intake (4 observational, 1 RCT). The review concluded that there is little evidence that maternal protein or carbohydrate intake affect offspring blood pressure [Brion *et al.*, 2008a].

208. Two further prospective studies in developed countries (not included in the review by Brion *et al* 2008a) have investigated the relationship between protein: carbohydrate ratio in the maternal diet and offspring blood pressure in adult life. These reported inconsistent findings: one showed a modest association [Roseboom *et al.*, 2001] but the other none [Huh *et al.*, 2005].

4.2.2.2   Birthweight and blood pressure

209. Most published studies have examined the relationship between birthweight alone and blood pressure, mainly in high income populations but occasionally in low income populations. Five systematic reviews of the birthweight-blood pressure

association have been identified [Law & Shiell, 1996; Huxley *et al.*, 2000; Huxley *et al.*, 2002; Schluchter, 2003; Gamborg, *et al.*, 2007].

210.   The most recent, a meta-analysis of birthweight and systolic blood pressure in adolescence and adulthood from 20 Nordic cohort studies (197,954 people born between 1910-1987), found an inverse association, irrespective of adjustment for current body mass index [Gamborg *et al.*, 2007]. At 50 years of age the estimated effect on systolic blood pressure was −1.52 mmHg/kg birthweight (95% CI −2.27, −0.77) in men and −2.80 mmHg/kg birthweight (95% CI −3.85, −1.76) in women. Publication bias was minimised by inclusion of published and unpublished studies, and no bias associated with strength of effect was identified. The association was stronger in the older age groups, and among females than males when limited to those with birthweight ≤4kg. The shape of the association was linear for males, but was inverted for females with a birthweight greater than 4kg.

211.   Another meta-analysis of observational studies published prior to 2000, included studies that provided quantitative estimates or reported on the direction of the association [Huxley *et al.*, 2002]. Of the 55 studies that reported a regression coefficient, 52 studies (95%) reported an inverse association.

212.   Meta-analyses of regression coefficients (involving 380,235 individuals) showed weaker associations among larger studies; −0.6mmHg/kg birthweight for more than about 3000 participants, −1.5mmHg/kg birthweight for 1000-3000 participants, and −1.9mmHg/kg birthweight for less than 1000 participants. This raises the possibility of publication bias towards preferential publication of small studies showing larger effects [Huxley *et al.*, 2002; Schluchter, 2003].

213.   The weaker associations observed in large studies could partly be explained if recall of birthweight were unreliable. Some of the studies (particularly those with at least 1000 participants) indeed relied on recall but most ascertained birthweight from contemporaneous records. Estimates of the effect size were similar in both types of study and this was also the case when the 17 largest studies (involving at least 1000 participants) were considered. There was no relationship between birthweight and age at blood pressure measurement, providing no evidence of altered effect size with age [Huxley *et al.*, 2002].

214.   The majority of studies included in the Huxley *et al.* (2002) meta-analysis were carried out in Europe and the USA, but findings were not appreciably different to those from Argentina, Brazil, China, Jamaica, and South Africa [Huxley *et al.*, 2002]. It nevertheless remains possible that birthweight explains some of the large differences in blood pressure between geographically dispersed populations [Marmot, 1984].

215.   Adjustment for current body weight (often used in earlier studies) appeared to amplify the association between birthweight and blood pressure by nearly a half (−0.6 mmHg/kg birthweight with adjustment for current weight, reduced to −0.4 mmHg/kg without adjustment) [Huxley *et al.*, 2002]. The inappropriateness of statistically adjusting the association between birthweight and blood pressure for current weight has been highlighted by others [Tu *et al.*, 2005].

216.   The estimate observed in 7 studies of monozygotic twin pairs was similar to that obtained in larger singleton studies with 1000 or more participants (−0.6mmHg/kg) but the relevance of twin studies to the developmental origins hypothesis [Symonds et al., 2000] is unclear since additional maternal and fetal adaptations may occur.

217.   A follow-up study of men and women born during 1935-43 found that an increase in placental:birthweight ratio was associated with an increase in adult blood pressure; mean systolic blood pressure rose by 15mmHg as placental weight increased from ≤1 lb to >1.5 lb and fell by 11mmHg as birthweight increased from ≤5.5 lb to >7.5 lb. The highest blood pressures were observed in individuals who had been small babies with large placentas [Barker et al., 1990].

218.   Overall, the epidemiological findings suggest that each 1kg increment in birthweight is associated with a reduction in blood pressure of under 2mmHg in later life [Huxley et al., 2000; Huxley et al., 2002]. However some have argued that this modest inverse association is of limited public health importance when compared to the magnitude of effects associated with later interventions [Huxley et al., 2002].

4.2.2.3   Early feeding and blood pressure

219.   A systematic review and meta-analysis of the association between infant feeding and blood pressure in later life identified 28 studies, all of which were observational (from both developed and developing countries), except one RCT of children who were premature at birth [Owen et al., 2003a]. Systolic blood pressure (SBP) was measured in infants, children and adults; the pooled mean difference in SBP was lower in those breastfed compared to those formula-fed (−1.10 mmHg, 95% CI −1.78, 0.42 mmHg), despite considerable heterogeneity between studies (p<0.001). Differences in diastolic blood pressure between breastfed and formula-fed infants were small; this finding was similar for studies of different sizes.

220.   Analysis to explain the source of heterogeneity showed that age group and length of gestation had no effect on SBP, though the size of effect decreased with increasing study size (Figure 9). The pooled estimate was larger in the 16 studies that reported the association between initial feeding and blood pressure in later life than in the 10 studies where data had been obtained by request. These findings raise the possibility of publication bias.

Figure 9 – Mean difference in systolic blood pressure between those breastfed versus formula-fed. Study author indicated on the y axis (as referenced in the original Owen et al., 2003a paper) in descending order of study size (N), grouped into studies with N>1000, N=300 to 1000, and N<300. Mean age (years) shown in parenthesis. Combined random effects estimate for each group shown by dashed vertical line and diamond (95% CI) [Owen et al., 2003a]

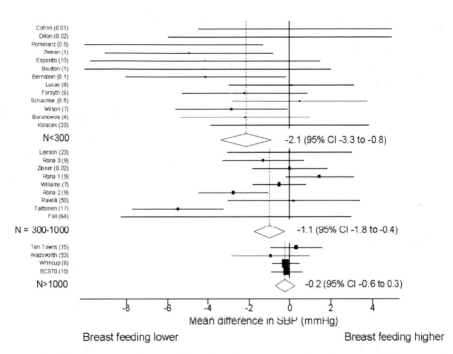

Reproduced with permission from Dr Christopher Owen, Division of Population Health Sciences and Education at St George's, University of London.

221.   Estimates of effects were similar in studies that recorded infant feeding status from contemporary records to those based on parental recall or self-report in later life. They were unaltered by adjustment for current body weight or size.

222.   The overall difference in SBP of 1.1 mmHg identified in the Owen et al (2003a) review seems modest but does not provide information about the effect of breastfeeding duration or exclusivity. These issues require further systematic examination in relevant studies. The definition of "breastfeeding" also requires more explicit definition in such reviews (see section 4.1.1).

223.   A further meta-analysis of the association between breastfeeding and blood pressure in later life [Martin et al., 2005b] included information from 15 studies (17,503 subjects) from the United Kingdom, Finland, Holland, Belgium, Italy, Czech Republic, Croatia, South Africa, and Australia. Three studies were not available at the time of the earlier review [Owen et al., 2003a] and two studies reported on follow-up into childhood, one into adulthood. Measurements in infancy and previously unpublished estimates used in the earlier meta-analysis [Owen et al., 2003a] were excluded, but a similar pooled difference in SBP was obtained (pooled difference −1.4 mmHg, 95% CI −2.2, −0.6). In the analyses, studies controlling

for socioeconomic factors showed smaller systolic blood pressure differences between breastfed and formula-fed subjects. The authors reported evidence of heterogeneity between study estimates.

224. The role of residual confounding in such studies is unclear, although two studies have shown that the association is independent of socioeconomic factors, maternal factors and anthropometric markers [Martin et al., 2004b; Lawlor et al., 2005].

225. Results from the Avon Longitudinal Study of Parents and Children (ALSPAC) found a positive association between sodium intake at 4 months and systolic blood pressure at 7 years (after minimal adjustment for child age, sex, energy[xxi]). Sodium intake (measured using diet diaries) at 4 months of 9 mmol per day was associated with an increase of 4.0mmHg in systolic blood pressure at 7 years. This was slightly attenuated after adjustment for breastfeeding [Brion et al., 2008b].

4.2.3   Blood cholesterol

4.2.3.1   Birthweight and blood cholesterol

226. The relationship between birthweight and adult blood cholesterol (mostly total cholesterol) has been examined in a number of narrative reviews, but 4 systematic reviews of the literature were identified [Lauren et al., 2003; Owen et al., 2003b; Huxley et al., 2004; Lawlor et al., 2006], one of which examined sex differences in the birthweight-blood cholesterol associations [Lawlor et al., 2006].

227. One of the systematic reviews included a meta-analysis of published regression coefficients examining the change in total cholesterol (TC) in a range of different age groups, associated with each 1kg increment in birthweight [Owen et al., 2003b]. Twenty-one out of 32 estimates (obtained from 28 studies in mostly developed countries, involving 23,247 individuals) showed an overall inverse association between birthweight and total blood cholesterol (Figure 10).

---

xxi   i.e. energy adjusted sodium intake, not absolute sodium intake.

Figure 10 – Regression coefficients for the change in total cholesterol (mmol/L) and 95% CI (horizontal lines) per 1 kg rise in birthweight for both males and females. Study author indicated on the y-axis (as referenced in the original Owen et al., 2003b paper) in ascending order of age (mean age shown in parenthesis). Combined estimate based on a random effects model [Owen et al., 2003b]

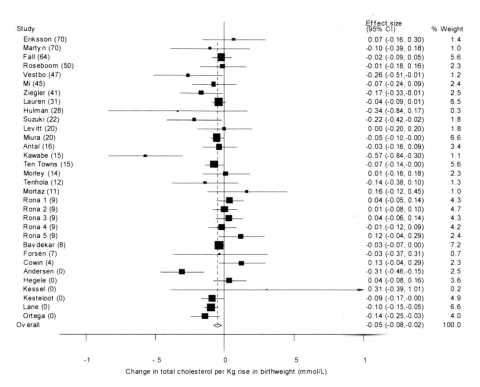

Study	Effect size (95% CI)	% Weight
Eriksson (70)	0.07 (-0.16, 0.30)	1.4
Martyn (70)	-0.10 (-0.39, 0.18)	1.0
Fall (64)	-0.02 (-0.09, 0.05)	5.6
Roseboom (50)	-0.01 (-0.18, 0.16)	2.3
Vestbo (47)	-0.26 (-0.51,-0.01)	1.2
Mi (45)	-0.07 (-0.24, 0.09)	2.4
Ziegler (41)	-0.17 (-0.33,-0.01)	2.5
Lauren (31)	-0.04 (-0.09, 0.01)	6.5
Hulman (28)	-0.34 (-0.84, 0.17)	0.3
Suzuki (22)	-0.22 (-0.42,-0.02)	1.8
Levitt (20)	0.00 (-0.20, 0.20)	1.8
Miura (20)	-0.05 (-0.10,-0.00)	6.6
Antal (16)	-0.03 (-0.16, 0.09)	3.4
Kawabe (15)	-0.57 (-0.84,-0.30)	1.1
Ten Towns (15)	-0.07 (-0.14,-0.00)	5.6
Morley (14)	0.01 (-0.16, 0.18)	2.3
Tenhola (12)	-0.14 (-0.38, 0.10)	1.3
Mortaz (11)	0.16 (-0.12, 0.45)	1.0
Rona 1 (9)	0.04 (-0.05, 0.14)	4.3
Rona 2 (9)	0.01 (-0.08, 0.10)	4.7
Rona 3 (9)	0.04 (-0.06, 0.14)	4.3
Rona 4 (9)	-0.01 (-0.12, 0.09)	4.2
Rona 5 (9)	0.12 (-0.04, 0.29)	2.4
Bavdekar (8)	-0.03 (-0.07, 0.00)	7.2
Forsén (7)	-0.03 (-0.37, 0.31)	0.7
Cowin (4)	0.13 (-0.04, 0.29)	2.3
Andersen (0)	-0.31 (-0.46,-0.15)	2.5
Hegele (0)	0.04 (-0.08, 0.16)	3.6
Kessel (0)	0.31 (-0.39, 1.01)	0.2
Kesteloot (0)	-0.09 (-0.17,-0.00)	4.9
Lane (0)	-0.10 (-0.15,-0.05)	6.6
Ortega (0)	-0.14 (-0.25,-0.03)	4.0
Overall	-0.05 (-0.08,-0.02)	100.0

Change in total cholesterol per Kg rise in birthweight (mmol/L)

228. The Owen et al (2003b) meta-analysis showed a fall of 0.05 mmol/L (95% CI −0.08, −0.02 mmol/L) in total cholesterol per kilogram rise in birthweight that was consistent between the sexes and different age groups. There was, however, a significant effect size difference between studies (test for heterogeneity between studies p<0.001). Unlike the birthweight-blood pressure relationship, adjustment for current body size and weight did not materially affect the overall estimate and there was little evidence of publication bias [Owen et al., 2003b].

229. A further review including both published and unpublished regression coefficients from 58 studies (with 68,974 individuals) alluded to the presence of publication bias and suggested that adjustment for current weight may unduly increase the inverse association between birthweight and blood cholesterol [Huxley et al., 2004]. However, an identical regression coefficient to the earlier meta-analysis was obtained (a −0.05 mmol/L fall in serum total cholesterol per kg rise in birthweight) [Huxley et al., 2004].

230. Meta-analysis by Lawlor et al (2006) included a total of 34 regression coefficients from 30 studies in developed countries, providing data on 33,650 males and 23,129

females. This observed a slightly stronger inverse association in males compared to females. The pooled within-study difference in age-adjusted regression coefficients was −0.03 mmol/l (CI −0.06, −0.01), and the pooled within-study difference in age and body mass index adjusted regression coefficients was −0.04 mmol/l (CI −0.07, −0.02).

231. The findings from these meta-analyses are consistent with those of a systematic review of 39 studies (involving 28,578 individuals including children, adolescents and adults) showing a modest association between birthweight and later serum lipid concentrations (including total cholesterol, low density lipoprotein, and high density lipoprotein) [Lauren et al., 2003].

232. In summary, the epidemiological data therefore suggest that there is a small inverse association between birthweight and later serum cholesterol concentration.

4.2.3.2 Early feeding and blood cholesterol

233. Two meta-analyses have examined the relationship between infant feeding and serum cholesterol in later life [Owen et al., 2002; Owen et al., 2008].

234. The first [Owen et al., 2002] identified 37 studies with 52 estimates (10,681 individuals including infants, children or adolescents, and adults) of total cholesterol (TC) concentration in those breastfed compared to those formula-fed. All were observational studies, mostly conducted in high-income populations (Figure 11). Mean TC in infancy was higher in breastfed than formula-fed infants (mean TC difference 0.64, 95% CI 0.50, 0.79 mmol/L), probably a consequence of the higher cholesterol content of breastmilk.

235. Mean TC in childhood and adolescence showed no consistent differences but in adults was generally lower in those who had been breastfed (mean TC difference −0.18, 95% CI −0.30, −0.06 mmol/L). Although the overall difference was modest (0.2 mmol/L) it was remarkably consistent between studies including subjects of different ages (from 17 to 64 years) and years of birth (from 1920 to 1975). This makes confounding by social circumstances unlikely, since the relation between social class and infant feeding has changed markedly during the 20th century. Persistence of the association after adjustment for social class was also demonstrated within individual studies [Marmot et al., 1980]. The findings were unchanged when the exclusiveness of feeding method (as defined by the study), or delay to maternal recall of feeding method were considered. Similar but weaker associations with LDL were evident throughout.

Figure 11 – Mean differences in total cholesterol (mmol/L) and 95% confidence intervals in infants, children, and adults, who were initially breastfed versus formula-fed (total cholesterol in those breastfed minus formula-fed). The box area is proportional to the inverse of the variance, with horizontal lines showing the 95% confidence intervals of the mean difference in cholesterol. The study author (as referenced in the original Owen et al., 2002 paper) is indicated on the y-axis in ascending age order. Males (M), females (F), all (A), and mean age (years) are shown in parenthesis. The combined estimate for each age group is shown by the dashed vertical line and diamond (95% CI) [Owen et al., 2002].

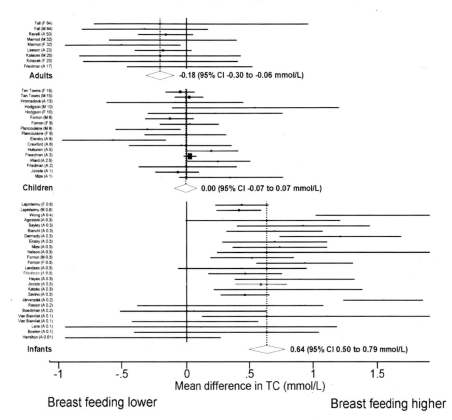

236.   The more recent review found that mean total blood cholesterol was 0.04mmol/L lower in adulthood (>16y) among those who were ever breastfed than among those who were fed formula (Figure 12) [Owen et al., 2008]. The difference was greater amongst studies that compared 'exclusive'[xxii] breastfeeding to formula feeding (Figure 13). Adjustment for potential confounders including socioeconomic position, body mass index, and smoking status in adults had minimal effect on these estimates.

xxii The author of the review defined exclusive breastfeeding by the WHO definition (i.e. breastfeeding while giving no other food or liquid), although few studies used this definition and exclusiveness of infant feeding was based on classification given in individual study reports, or where applicable, reported directly by the author.

Figure 12 – Mean (and 95% CI) differences in blood cholesterol in breastfed versus bottle-fed participants in 17 studies (16 crude estimates, 1 adjusted for age). The box area of each study is proportional to the inverse of the variance, and the horizontal lines show the 95% CI. First author (and reference number) as cited in the original Owen *et al.*, 2008 paper, is listed on the y-axis; mean age is shown in ascending order; "M" refers to male-only studies. The pooled estimate based on a fixed-effects model is shown by a dashed vertical line and ◊ (95% CI) [Owen *et al.*, 2008].

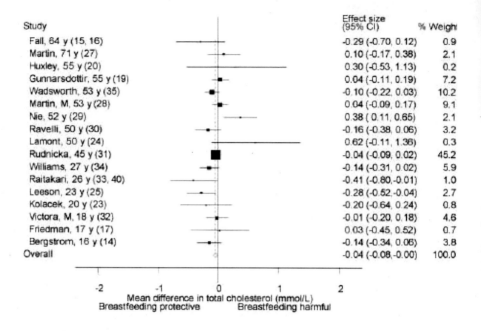

Study	Effect size (95% CI)	% Weight
Fall, 64 y (15, 16)	-0.29 (-0.70, 0.12)	0.9
Martin, 71 y (27)	0.10 (-0.17, 0.38)	2.1
Huxley, 55 y (20)	0.30 (-0.53, 1.13)	0.2
Gunnarsdottir, 55 y (19)	0.04 (-0.11, 0.19)	7.2
Wadsworth, 53 y (35)	-0.10 (-0.22, 0.03)	10.2
Martin, M, 53 y (28)	0.04 (-0.09, 0.17)	9.1
Nie, 52 y (29)	0.38 (0.11, 0.65)	2.1
Ravelli, 50 y (30)	-0.16 (-0.38, 0.06)	3.2
Lamont, 50 y (24)	0.62 (-0.11, 1.36)	0.3
Rudnicka, 45 y (31)	-0.04 (-0.09, 0.02)	45.2
Williams, 27 y (34)	-0.14 (-0.31, 0.02)	5.9
Raitakari, 26 y (33, 40)	-0.41 (-0.80, -0.01)	1.0
Leeson, 23 y (25)	-0.28 (-0.52, -0.04)	2.7
Kolacek, 20 y (23)	-0.20 (-0.64, 0.24)	0.8
Victora, M, 18 y (32)	-0.01 (-0.20, 0.18)	4.6
Friedman, 17 y (17)	0.03 (-0.45, 0.52)	0.7
Bergstrom, 16 y (14)	-0.14 (-0.34, 0.06)	3.8
Overall	-0.04 (-0.08, -0.00)	100.0

Mean difference in total cholesterol (mmol/L)
Breastfeeding protective   Breastfeeding harmful

Reproduced from: Am J Clin Nutr (2008, vol 88(2), pages 305-314) with permission from American Society for Nutrition.

Figure 13 – Mean (and 95% CI) differences in blood cholesterol in breastfed versus bottle-fed participants in 7 studies that reported exclusive breastfeeding or bottle-feeding in early life. The box area of each study is proportional to the inverse of the variance, and the horizontal lines show the 95% CI. First author (and reference number) as cited in the original Owen et al., 2008 paper, and mean age (y) is given in ascending order. The pooled estimate based on a fixed-effects model is shown by a dashed vertical line and ◊ (95% CI) [Owen et al., 2008].

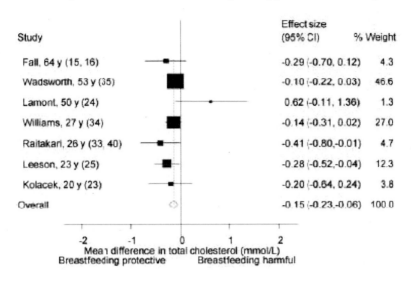

Reproduced from: Am J Clin Nutr (2008, vol 88(2), pages 305-314) with permission from American Society for Nutrition.

237.   Overall, the epidemiological data show that formula-fed infants have lower blood cholesterol levels initially; however adults who were breastfed, particularly if exclusively breastfed, have lower blood cholesterol concentrations than those who were not breastfed. The mechanism is unclear but it has been hypothesised that early life exposure to breastmilk may lead to reduced cholesterol synthesis in later life.

4.2.4   Other cardiovascular outcomes

4.2.4.1   Birthweight and other cardiovascular outcomes

238.   Lower birthweight has been related to haemorrhagic stroke [Hypponen et al., 2001], atherosclerotic changes [Martyn et al., 1998; Gale et al., 2002] and adverse haemostatic profile (including elevated levels of serum fibrinogen) [Barker & Martyn, 1992], although these associations have not always been found [Tilling et al., 2004]. Compared to the number of studies relating birthweight to coronary heart disease, too few have examined the association with other cardiovascular outcomes for the consistency of associations to be evaluated.

4.3 Body composition

4.3.1 Birthweight and later body composition

239. The majority of studies have examined associations between birthweight and later BMI as an indicator of adiposity. Two systematic reviews [Parsons *et al.*, 1999; Rogers, 2003] of studies in mainly developed countries have concluded that there is a positive association between birthweight, attained BMI and prevalence of obesity (as defined by BMI) in later life. The association was strongest in children and young adults but weakened in middle aged adults [Rogers, 2003]. Heterogeneity in the presentation of results obviated meta-analysis but two additional studies have estimated that a 1 kg increment in birthweight is associated with a 0.5 to 0.7 kg/m² rise in the BMI of young adults [Sorensen *et al.*, 1997; Loos *et al.*, 2001].

240. Some studies suggest that both low and high birthweight are associated with subsequent obesity risk in young adults and children (as defined using BMI), implying a J-shaped or U-shaped relationship [Rogers, 2003]. The confounding influence of parental BMI, however, needs to be established, as this could account for the positive association observed between high birthweight and subsequent BMI.

241. Few studies have explored the relationship between birthweight and measures of body composition other than BMI. One review observed inconsistent associations [Wells *et al.*, 2007a]. In this review, one study of over 6,000 9–10 year old children observed that birthweight was positively correlated with both lean body mass and total body fat (assessed by dual-energy x-ray absorptiometry) after adjustment for current height. Some studies cited in this review indicated that relationships with ponderal index at birth were even stronger.

242. One study included in the Wells *et al* (2007) review examined the relationship between birthweight and body composition at birth in Indian neonates relative to babies in the UK [Yajnik *et al.*, 2003]. The Indian neonates showed much reduced birthweight and waist circumference, but more modest deficits in skinfold thickness, especially on the trunk. The Indian neonates had reduced lean mass, but truncal fat formed a higher proportion of fat mass at birth.

243. Compared with UK adults, the average adult from India of similar height and weight also has a greater fat mass and greater central fat distribution [Yajnik, 2002]. This is associated with increased risk of heart disease and metabolic syndrome. The presence of this pattern of body composition at birth suggests that it cannot be entirely attributed to aspects of diet or lifestyle during adulthood [Yajnik *et al.*, 2003].

244. A retrospective study (included in the Wells *et al* 2007a review) of older adults born in Hertfordshire reported an increased percentage fat mass, total and central fat mass after adjusting for adult BMI in those who were of low birthweight (mean 2.76 kg), relative to those of high birthweight (mean 4.23 kg) [Kensara *et al.*, 2005]. Low birthweight subjects are also shown to have lower energy expenditure [Kensara *et al.*, 2006] which may be related to their lower fat-free mass (FFM). Adjusting for adult BMI however leaves doubt as to whether the association of

birthweight with low lean body mass was truly programmed before birth [Wells *et al.*, 2007a] or whether growth patterns induced by factors operating between birth and follow-up are more responsible [Lucas *et al.*, 1999].

245. A cross-sectional study of 8,760 adults born in Helsinki, published since the Wells *et al* (2007a) review, found that birthweight was significantly correlated with lean body mass but not fat mass (a 1 kg increase in birthweight corresponded in men to a 4.1 kg increase in adult lean mass (95% CI 3.1, 5.1) and in women to a 2.9 kg (95% CI 2.1, 3.6) increase). This association was unaffected after adjustment for age, adult body size, physical activity, smoking status, social class and maternal size [Yliharsila *et al.*, 2007]. The association between birthweight and later BMI may not therefore reflect truly increased adiposity [Rogers, 2003]. Another study in children observed a significant positive association between birthweight and height (explaining an increasing proportion of the variability up to 5 years of age (r^2 =0.194; r =0.440; p=0.001) and decreasing thereafter (r^2 =0.103 at 7.8 years of age; r=0.320; p=0.003). Childhood fat mass was negatively associated with birthweight (an increase in birthweight of 1 standard deviation (SD) was associated with a decrease of 1.95% fat (p=0.012) and independent of a number of factors adjusted for [Elia *et al.*, 2007].

246. In summary, there is evidence that higher birthweight is associated with higher BMI in later life though there remains some doubt about what BMI reflects in terms of body composition in this context. The few studies of body composition that have been able to resolve separately the fat and lean mass components suggest that higher birthweight may later be associated with relatively greater lean mass, whereas lower birthweight is associated later with relatively greater fat mass. However, this does not necessarily confirm a direct link between birthweight and central fat distribution.

4.3.2 Postnatal growth and body composition

247. Observational studies in industrialised countries have also associated rapid infancy weight gain with later obesity (defined by BMI or skinfold thickness) in childhood and adulthood [Stettler, 2007]. This has also been associated with an increase in fat mass, adjusted for height.

248. A systematic review of 22 cohort and two case-control studies (mostly based in developed countries) [Baird *et al.*, 2005] concluded that those who were at the highest end of the distribution for weight or BMI in infancy, or those who grow rapidly during infancy, were at increased risk of subsequent obesity (defined by BMI) as children and adults.

249. Two further systematic reviews of studies mainly from developed countries have examined the relationship between rapid weight gain in infancy and later obesity [Monteiro & Victora, 2005; Ong & Loos, 2006]. The first indicated that rapid growth during the first years of life is associated with the prevalence of obesity later in life [Monteiro & Victora, 2005]. The most recent [Ong & Loos, 2006], which identified 21 studies, also concluded that there is a strong association between rapid weight gain in infancy and later risk of obesity. Subsequently published results from cross

sectional [Dennison *et al.*, 2006] and longitudinal studies [Dubois & Girard, 2006; Karaolis-Danckett *et al.*, 2006] have confirmed these conclusions.

250. It has been suggested that associations between infant weight gain and later body composition may vary between developed and developing countries [Wells *et al.*, 2007a]. Studies suggest that infant weight gain is positively associated with weight, height and lean mass, but only those conducted in developed countries have found a positive association specifically with adult fat mass [Li *et al.*, 2003; Wells & Victora, 2005]. This may reflect a need for infants in developing countries to direct energy towards reducing deficits in lean mass present at birth, whereas in developed countries additional energy is stored as fat mass.

251. The impact of postnatal growth on later body composition is not restricted to infancy. Rapid weight gain during childhood is also associated with increased risk of obesity later, as defined by BMI [Cole, 2004a].

4.3.3   Early feeding and later body composition

252. Two meta-analyses suggest that breastfeeding, relative to formula feeding, is associated with a decreased risk of later obesity [Arenz *et al.*, 2004; Owen *et al.*, 2005]. The first was a systematic review and meta-analysis of nine published epidemiological studies, all from developed countries, and included >69,000 individuals (analysis included children 5 and 18 years) [Arenz *et al.*, 2004]. It showed that breastfeeding reduced the risk of obesity[xxiii] in childhood significantly (adjusted OR 0.78, 95% CI 0.71, 0.85) and this was unaffected by adjustment of a number of confounders. A second meta-analysis [Owen *et al.*, 2005] identifying 28 studies (4 in infants, 23 in children and 2 in adults and a total of 298,900 subjects) also reported a reduced risk of obesity[xxiv] (OR: 0.87 95% CI 0.85, 0.89). Both studies identified categorical and dose-response effects.

253. Another meta-analysis of studies based in developed countries also observed an inverse dose-response association between duration of breastfeeding and risk of overweight, as categorised by BMI (no definition of overweight was used) [Harder *et al.*, 2005] (Figure 14). Up to 9 months' duration, each month of breastfeeding was associated with a 4% decrease in risk (OR 0.96 per month of breastfeeding, 95% CI 0.94, 0.98). However, the association between early feeding and later body size may be influenced by confounding factors, such as maternal body size, maternal smoking and socio-demographic factors.

---

xxiii Studies included in the systematic review used different percentiles for the definition of obesity, but the author reports the results were comparable and the sensitivity analysis showed no difference between a cutoff at the 90th, 95th and 97th percentile.

xxiv The definitions of obesity differed among studies included in this meta-analysis, largely depending on the age at measurement. Most studies used a percentile cutoff based on BMI, describing subjects at the tail of the distribution. The 95th or 97th percentile was used most often, although some studies used cutoff values as low as the 85th percentile [Owen et al., 2005].

Figure 14 – Odds ratios (with corresponding 95% confidence intervals in parentheses) for overweight, per month of breastfeeding. Studies are ordered alphabetically by first author (as referenced in the original Harder *et al.*, 2005 paper). The pooled or "combined" odds ratio (OR) was calculated [Harder *et al.*, 2005].

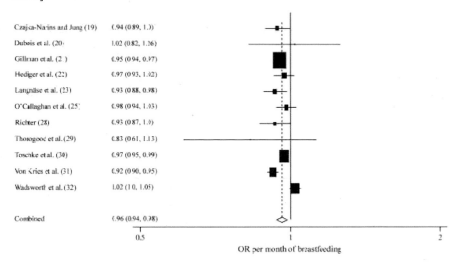

Reproduced from: Harder T *et al.*, Duration of breastfeeding and risk of overweight: a meta-analysis, Am J Epidemiol, 2005, vol 162, pages 397-403 with permission from Oxford University Press.

254.   The Southampton Women's Survey (SWS) found a statistically significant association between longer duration of breastfeeding and lower fat mass at 4 years (measured by DXA). The fat mass in children breastfed for 12 months or more was 4.5 kg (95% CI 4.3, 4.7 kg), compared with 5.0 kg (95% CI 4.7, 5.3 kg) in children never breastfed. This was unaffected by adjustment for confounders including a range of maternal factors, infant birthweight and age of introduction of solids [Robinson *et al.*, 2009]. There was a weak inverse association (p=0.034) between age of introduction of solid foods and fat mass at 4 years of age, but this disappeared after adjustment for confounders. No associations were found with BMI, but overweight and obese children[xxv] tended to be breastfed for shorter periods. Other studies that have measured fat mass and fat-free mass, have not confirmed a reduced risk of adiposity, where no association was observed after adjustment for confounders [Victora *et al.*, 2003; Toschke *et al.*, 2007].

4.4   Diabetes and glucose intolerance

4.4.1   Birthweight, glucose intolerance and diabetes

255.   Three narrative reviews of literature relating birthweight to diabetic risk factors or type 2 diabetes were identified [Holness *et al.*, 2000; Bertram & Hanson, 2001; Byrne, 2001]. Two systematic reviews (one with meta-analysis) have also examined the association between birthweight and diabetes or impaired glucose tolerance

---

xxv according to the International Obesity Taskforce cut-offs for overweight and obesity.

in adult life [Newsome *et al.*, 2003; Whincup *et al.*, 2008]. Most of the studies identified were performed in developed countries.

256. Most of the studies identified in the first review [Newsome *et al.*, 2003] reported inverse associations between birthweight and markers of diabetes; 15 out of 25 (60%) showed an inverse association with fasting plasma glucose, 20 out of 26 (77%) with fasting plasma insulin, and 13 out of 16 (81%) with the prevalence of type 2 diabetes. The inverse associations reported were not explained by inter-study differences in gender, age, or current weight and BMI. The authors did not attempt meta-analysis.

257. Results from the most recent meta-analytic review [Whincup *et al.*, 2008] are nevertheless consistent with these findings. Low birthweight (<2.5 kg) was associated with an increased risk of type 2 diabetes: 23 out of 31 studies reported inverse associations between birthweight and type 2 diabetes associations. In nine they were statistically significant. The inverse pattern of association extended to birthweights of at least 3 kg, although the authors could not exclude a modest positive association between birthweight and type 2 diabetes for birthweights exceeding 4 kg. Overall each 1 kg increment in birthweight was associated with a 20% reduction in the odds of later developing type 2 diabetes (OR 0.80, 95% CI 0.72, 0.89). Adjustment for socioeconomic status did not affect the association but adjustment for current body mass index slightly strengthened it.

258. The review by Whincup *et al* (2008) indicated that in all populations, excluding North American Indians and one group of White Canadians, the relationship between birthweight and adult type 2 diabetes risk is strongly inverse. There was no firm evidence of publication bias.

259. Another meta-analysis also observed an association between low birthweight (<2500g) and increased risk of type 2 diabetes in adults (OR 1.32, 95% CI 1.06, 1.64). However in this study a similar increase in risk (OR 1.27, 95% CI 1.01, 1.59) was attributable to birthweight exceeding 4000g compared with birthweight <4000g [Harder *et al.*, 2007]. Thus overall a U-shaped relationship was identified.

260. There is a well-established association between the peroxisome proliferator-activated receptor (PPAR)-γ2 gene and type 2 diabetes. In people of low birthweight, the Pro12Pro polymorphism of the PPAR-γ2 gene has been shown to be associated with increased insulin resistance, and elevated plasma insulin concentrations in later life [Eriksson *et al.*, 2002]. This association was not observed in people with normal birthweights suggesting that the fetal environment interacts with the effects of the PPAR-γ2 Pro12Ala polymorphism to modify the expression of PPAR-γ2 later in life.

261. The relationship between type 1 diabetes and birthweight has been less frequently studied though a meta-analytic review identified increased risk among those of higher birthweight [Harder *et al.*, 2009]. This observation was questioned on grounds of reported publication bias, unsatisfactory adjustment for confounders and inclusion of duplicate cases [Cardwell & Patterson 2009].

262. In summary, the epidemiological evidence suggests that lower birthweight is associated with greater risk of impaired glucose tolerance or type 2 diabetes in later life. This finding is consistent with the observation that lower birthweight is associated with relatively greater fat than lean mass in later life.

4.4.2 Postnatal growth, glucose intolerance and diabetes

263. Risk for many aspects of metabolic syndrome appears greatest in those born small who subsequently gain the most weight [Bavdekar et al., 1999; Barker et al., 2002].

264. A longitudinal study of 8,760 subjects born in Helsinki (1934-1944) showed that type 2 diabetes in adult life was associated with earlier adiposity rebound[xxvi]. The risk of later type 2 diabetes fell from 8.6% in those showing adiposity rebound before the age of 5 years to 1.8% among those in whom it occurred after 7 years of age. Earlier adiposity rebound was preceded by low ponderal index at birth (p<0.001), low BMI at 1 year of age, low weight at 1 year and low weight velocity during infancy. Current BMI of these subjects was not known [Eriksson et al., 2003].

265. The early life growth patterns of individuals in this cohort who later developed coronary heart disease (CHD) resembled the growth patterns preceding type 2 diabetes. Both groups showed lower birthweight and thinness at 1 year of age, followed by the attainment of higher body mass index later in childhood. Most subjects who developed type 2 diabetes in this cohort were not obese during childhood [Eriksson, 2006].

266. Early adiposity rebound in the 1946 British birth cohort was also associated with significantly increased risk of type 2 diabetes at 31 to 53 years of age. The association was independent of birthweight but slightly attenuated by adjustment for sex and adult height (p=0.003). It was not statistically significant after adjustment for sex and adult BMI (p=0.1), or further adjustment for birthweight, weight at 2 years, adult height, social class and parental diabetes (p=0.4) [Wadsworth et al., 2005].

267. A prospective, population-based study in India observed an association between thinness in infancy and impaired glucose tolerance or diabetes in young adult life [Bhargava et al., 2004]. Glucose tolerance and plasma insulin concentrations were measured in 1492 men and women aged 26 to 32 years, who had been measured at birth and at intervals of 3 to 6 months throughout infancy, childhood, and adolescence. Impaired glucose tolerance or diabetes was associated with low BMI up to the age of 2 years, followed by an early adiposity rebound and accelerated increase in BMI until adulthood. However, none of the subjects were obese at age 12 years.

4.4.3 Early feeding, glucose intolerance and diabetes

268. A meta-analysis examining the influence of initial breastfeeding on type 2 diabetes, and blood glucose and insulin concentrations [Owen et al., 2006], observed that breastfeeding in infancy (relative to formula feeding) was associated with a modest reduction in risk of type 2 diabetes (OR 0.61 95% CI 0.44, 0.85). The

---

xxvi Early adiposity rebound – the early age-related fall in BMI was followed by an increase before 6 years of age, the average (SD) in this study being 5.8 (1.0) years [Eriksson et al, 2003].

analysis incorporated 7 studies (3 conducted in North America and 4 in Europe) which recruited 76,744 subjects. Amongst non-diabetic subjects those who were breastfed showed lower fasting insulin concentrations in later life.

269. Studies of Pima Indians in the US and those born around the time of the Dutch Famine (1943-1947) have shown that those breastfed (according to contemporaneous feeding records) have less insulin resistance and glucose intolerance than those formula-fed [Pettitt et al., 1997; Ravelli et al., 2000]. A small case-control study of Native Canadians showed that those breastfed were at lower risk of type 2 diabetes in childhood [Young et al., 2002], although bias in the recall of infant feeding practices by parental or caregiver interview cannot be excluded.

270. Overall, the epidemiological evidence suggests that infants who are not breastfed are at greater risk of type 2 diabetes in later life.

271. A short duration of breastfeeding and early introduction of cow's milk have been reported to be associated with an increased risk of type 1 diabetes [Borch-Johnsen et al., 1984; Gerstein, 1994] and it has been hypothesised that breastmilk may protect against early development of type 1 diabetes [Schrezenmeir & Jagla, 2000; Shehadeh et al., 2001].

272. Associations between type 1 diabetes and infant feeding method have mainly been observed in childhood case-control studies utilising retrospective ascertainment of infant feeding practices [Visalli et al., 2003; EURODIAB Substudy 2 Study Group, 2002]. This raises the possibility of recall bias, an explanation supported by further meta-analysis of 17 case-control studies demonstrating little effect in studies based on contemporaneous feeding records [Norris & Scott, 1996]. More recent studies that have included a prospective nested case-control design have similarly failed to observe an effect [Thorsdottir et al., 2000; Virtanen et al., 2000]. Overall there is little current evidence to support an effect of infant feeding method on the pathogenesis of type 1 diabetes.

4.5   Cancer

4.5.1   Child leukaemia

4.5.1.1   Maternal nutrient intake and child leukaemia

273. A case-control study in Western Australia observed a 60% reduced risk of acute lymphocytic leukaemia (ALL) in the offspring of mothers who took iron and folate supplements in pregnancy. Births between 1984 and 1992 were studied, including 83 children with acute lymphocytic leukaemia, and 166 controls of matched background (subjects were aged 0 to 14 years). The reduced risk appeared principally attributable to folate intake since consumption of iron supplements alone was associated with a reduced risk of only 25% [Thompson et al.; 2001].

4.5.1.2   Birthweight and child leukaemia

274.   High birthweight has been associated with increased risk of childhood leukaemia. A meta-analysis identified 18 studies (15 case-control; 2 "case-referent"[xxvii] and 1 cohort study) including 10,282 children with leukaemia [Hjalgrim *et al.*, 2003]. Those with birthweight of 4kg or more had a higher risk of ALL than those who weighed less than 4kg (OR 1.26, 95% CI 1.17, 1.37) and a graded effect was observed (see Figure 15). Similarly a graded increase in risk of acute myeloid leukaemia (AML) was observed among children weighing 4,000 g or more at birth (OR 1.27, 95% CI 0.73, 2.20) but there was considerable variation between study results.

Figure 15 – Study-specific crude odds ratios for leukaemia, per 1kg increase in birthweight for acute lymphoblastic leukaemia (ALL) and leukaemia combined (author listed as referenced by Hjalgrim *et al.*, 2003) [Hjalgrim *et al.*, 2003].

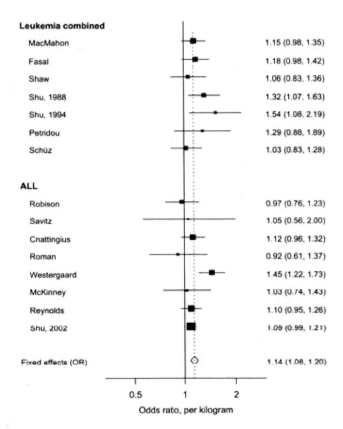

Reproduced from: Hjalgrim LL *et al.*, Birth weight as a risk factor for childhood leukemia: a meta-analysis of 18 epidemiologic studies, Am J Epidemiol, 2003, vol 158, pages 724-735, with permission from Oxford University Press.

275.   A population-based, case-control study (3,812 cases) in Denmark, Sweden, Norway, and Iceland noted that risk of ALL but not AML was positively associated with birthweight [Hjalgrim *et al.*, 2004]. A prospective study in Israel (n=86,604; 65

---

xxvii Birthweights of cases were compared with birthweight reference data.

cases of childhood leukaemia) observed a positive linear relationship between birthweight and both AML and ALL [Paltiel et al., 2004].

276.   A cohort of 576,593 infants born in Australia were followed from birth to examine the relation between birthweight, intrauterine growth, and risk of childhood leukaemia (243 cases ALL and 36 cases AML). Cases were followed up from birth to diagnosis, and noncases were followed up from birth to either the child's 15th birthday, the child's date of death, or to the end of the follow-up period, whichever came first [Milne et al., 2007]. Risk of ALL was positively associated with the proportion of "optimal" birthweight achieved[xxviii]. The effect was strongest among children younger than 5 years, in whom the association was not altered by excluding high birthweight (defined as >3,500 g, >3,800 g and >4,000 g) babies.

277.   In summary, the epidemiological evidence (primarily from case control studies) consistently indicates that greater birthweight is associated with increased risk of ALL but there is inconsistent evidence of a relationship with AML.

4.5.1.3   Early feeding and childhood cancers

278.   A meta-analysis of 24 case control studies and 2 cohort/nested case-control studies, mainly from developed countries, observed a lower risk of childhood cancer amongst those who had been breastfed. The pooled ORs for breastfed infants, as opposed to those never breastfed, were 0.91 (95% CI 0.84, 0.98) for acute lymphoblastic leukaemia, 0.76 (95% CI 0.60, 0.97) for Hodgkin's disease and 0.59 (95% CI 0.44, 0.78) for neuroblastoma [Martin et al., 2005a]. Eighty five per cent of the studies relied on long-term recall of feeding history and exclusivity of breastfeeding was examined in only 8% of the studies.

4.5.2   Breast cancer

4.5.2.1   Birthweight, size at birth and breast cancer

279.   The most recent meta-analysis of the relationship between birthweight, size at birth and breast cancer (including 32 studies from developed countries and a total 22,508 breast cancer cases, both pre and postmenopausal) found moderate positive associations in studies based on birth records [dos Santos Silva et al., 2008]. The risk of breast cancer rose with increasing birthweight, length and head circumference. A 0.5kg increment in birthweight was associated with a significant increase in risk (pooled RR 1.06, 95% CI 1.02, 1.09; p=0.002). Women who were ≥51 cm long at birth showed a 17% (95% CI 2 to 35%) greater risk of developing breast cancer relative to those in the baseline category for length (49.0 – 49.9cm), whilst those who had a head circumference at birth of ≥35 cm had an 11% increase (95% CI –5% to 29%) in risk relative to those in the baseline category for head circumference (33.0 – 33.9 cm). These effects were not confounded by known breast cancer risk factors (including maternal age, maternal parity and maternal birth size) nor moderated by age or menopausal status.

---

xxviii "Optimal birthweight" was calculated by adjusting birthweight for gestation, maternal height, parity, and infant sex, and comparing this to that expected in a population of singleton births with no recorded pathological factors constraining fetal growth, including maternal smoking [Blair et al., 2005].

280. A review including 4 cohort and 12 case-control studies investigating the association between several early life exposures and breast cancer [Forman et al., 2005] showed that heavier babies (birthweight ≥4000g) experienced an increased risk of premenopausal breast cancer compared to those of lower weight (2500-2999g). Evidence relating to postmenopausal breast cancer was inconsistent. Amongst studies in which birth length was positively associated with breast cancer risk the effect size was greater than for birthweight alone. A systematic review by Okasha et al. (2003) which investigated the influence of a number of early life exposures, also concluded that there was evidence of a positive relationship between birthweight and breast cancer, primarily from cohort studies.

281. The World Cancer Research Fund systematic review identified 6 cohort studies and 4 case-control studies, concluding that greater birthweight 'probably' increases risk of premenopausal breast cancer. Meta-analysis of the cohort data showed an 8 percent increase in risk per kilogram of birthweight (OR 1.08, 95% CI 1.04, 1.13) [World Cancer Research Fund / American Institute for Cancer Research, 2007]. No association was found between birthweight and postmenopausal breast cancer.

282. A study of 475 women born around the 1944-1945 Dutch famine has shown that those exposed to famine in utero more frequently reported breast cancer than unexposed women. The birthweights of women with breast cancer (mean 3191g) did not differ significantly from those of women without breast cancer (mean 3296g). The effect was largest, and statistically significant, among women who were conceived during the famine [Painter et al., 2006]. Roseboom et al. (2006) also found that women exposed to famine early in fetal life were at increased risk of breast cancer.

283. In summary, there is consistent evidence that larger babies are at greater risk of breast cancer, particularly premenopausal breast cancer. However, birthweight itself does not capture the complexity of the relationship. Where studied, length at birth appears to exert a stronger effect than weight, emphasising the importance of distinguishing between birthweight, size and body composition.

4.5.2.2 Postnatal growth and breast cancer

284. Greater body fatness during childhood and adolescence has been associated with decreased incidence of premenopausal and postmenopausal breast cancer in several retrospective and prospective studies [Le Marchand et al., 1988; Berkey et al., 1999; Hilakivi-Clarke et al., 2001; Ahlgren et al., 2004; Weiderpass et al., 2004; De Stavola et al., 2004; Baer et al., 2005]. No systematic review or meta-analysis was identified.

285. A prospective study of Danish women (n=117,415; 3,340 cases) found independent risk factors for breast cancer (representing both pre and postmenopausal cancers) included early age at peak growth velocity, tall stature at 14 years of age, low BMI at 14 years of age and high growth rate in childhood, particularly around puberty (8 to 14 years of age) [Ahlgren et al., 2004].

286. A British cohort study following 2,176 girls for 55 years identified 57 cases of breast cancer (including both pre and postmenopausal cancers). Risk was increased amongst those showing fastest growth in height between 4-7 years (OR 1.54 per SD increase in height velocity, 95% CI 1.13, 2.09) and between 11-15 years (OR 1.29 per SD of height velocity, 95% CI 0.97, 1.71). In contrast, risk decreased with greater body mass index velocity at age 2-4 years (OR 0.63 per SD increase in BMI velocity, 95% CI 0.48, 0.83). These effects were most marked in women who attained menarche before the age of 12.5 years [De Stavola et al., 2004].

287. A cohort study of 3,447 women born in Helsinki found that women developing postmenopausal breast cancer later in life were on average taller and had lower BMI at each age from 7-15 years (p<0.05 at each age) [Hilakivi-Clarke et al., 2001]. Another prospective study of 99,717 women in Norway and Sweden found an association with premenopausal cancer, where women taller than 160cm had a 30% increased risk compared with shorter individuals, but there was no evidence for a linear association [Weiderpass et al., 2004].

288. A matched case-control study nested in an historical cohort of 30,084 women born in Hawaii [Le Marchand et al., 1988], found a statistically significant negative association between adolescent body mass (girls aged 10-14 years) and premenopausal breast cancer (p=0.004). This association was strongest in those overweight who remained overweight in adulthood. Early age weight, height and body surface area were not associated with pre- or postmenopausal cancer.

289. Analysis of 65,140 women in the Nurse's Health Study found that later menarche (RR 0.52 for ≥15 years vs. ≤11 years) and more body fatness at age 10 years (RR 0.60 for fattest vs. leanest) were associated with a decreased risk of premenopausal breast carcinoma. These associations remained after adjustment for a number of confounders [Berkey et al., 1999].

290. Analysis of 109,267 premenopausal women from the Nurse's Health Study II found an inverse association between body fatness at age 5, 10 and 20 years and premenopausal breast cancer (RRs 0.48, 95% CI 0.35, 0.55 and RR 0.57, 95% CI 0.39, 0.83 for the most overweight compared with the most lean in childhood and adolescence, respectively). The association for childhood body fatness was slightly attenuated after adjustment for later BMI (RR 0.52, 95% CI 0.38, 0.71) [Baer et al., 2005].

291. In summary, taller height[xxix] during childhood and adolescence and faster than average height growth are associated with an increased risk of premenopausal breast cancer in later life. Conversely, greater body fatness during childhood and adolescence is associated with a reduced risk of breast cancer in later life (particularly premenopausal breast cancer).

4.5.2.3 Early feeding and breast cancer

292. A meta-analysis of 8 case-control and 3 cohort/nested case-control studies included 11,564 breast cancer cases but found no association between overall risk

---

xxix Attained height is often interpreted as a marker for rate of growth.

of breast cancer and ever being breastfed [Martin et al., 2005d]. Sub-analysis of the 3,347 cases of premenopausal breast cancer in 9 studies however identified some reduction in risk associated with ever being breastfed (RR 0.88, 95% CI 0.79, 0.98).

4.5.3   Colorectal cancer

4.5.3.1   Birthweight, length at birth and colorectal cancer

293.   A British prospective study of 11,857 individuals observed a J-shaped relationship between self-reported birthweight and subsequent risk of colorectal cancer in both men and women [Sandhu et al., 2002]. Relative to a reference group weighing 2500-3249g, the age and sex adjusted hazard ratio for people born with birthweight ›4000g was 2.57 (95% CI 1.15, 5.74). There was also evidence that low birthweight babies (‹2500g) were at increased risk compared to the reference group.

294.   A prospective study of 35,697 people in Norway, using registry data on birthweight and size, observed a higher risk of colorectal cancer (RR 1.9, 95% CI 1.0, 3.7) in men with shorter birth length [Nilsen et al., 2005a]. Similar associations were found for birthweight and head circumference, but among women there was no association with birthweight or any other dimensions.

295.   The evidence associating birthweight and risk of colorectal cancer is therefore inconclusive at present.

4.5.4   Prostate cancer

4.5.4.1   Birthweight, size and body composition at birth and prostate cancer

296.   A Swedish study identified 21 cases among 366 men of known birthweight who had been recruited to a cohort study in 1913. The incidence of prostate cancer was about five times higher in the highest quartile of birthweight than in other birthweight groups: incidence was 6.00 per 1,000 person years in the highest percentile category (which had median birthweight 4850g) compared to 1.07 in the lowest category (median birthweight 2640g) [Tibblin et al., 1995].

297.   However, no association between birthweight and total prostate cancer risk was observed in a retrospective cohort study in the USA (n=21,140) [Platz et al., 1998] and a prospective study in Norway (n=19,681) [Nilsen et al., 2005b]. In the US study, a slight elevation in risk of high stage/grade tumours was seen at higher birthweights, but the relationship was not linear [Platz et al., 1998]. The Norwegian study observed that among a subset of men who presented with metastatic prostate cancer those in the highest quartile of birth length (≥53cm) were at greater risk than men in the lowest quartile (less than 51 cm). However, there was no trend across the distribution of birth length [Nilsen et al., 2005b].

298.   A Swedish population-based nested case-control study (250 cases; 691 controls) observed no significant association between birth size or placental weight and prostate cancer risk [Ekbom et al., 1996]. However, ponderal index (kg/m^3) at birth was associated with an increased risk of death from prostate cancer. A further

population-based nested case-control study in Sweden (834 cases; 1,880 controls) found birthweight, birth length, and placental weight to be unrelated to prostate cancer risk [Ekbom *et al.*, 2000].

299. The evidence supporting an association between birthweight and risk of prostate cancer is inconclusive.

4.5.5 Oesophageal and gastric cancer

4.5.5.1 Birthweight and oesophageal or gastric cancer

300. A prospective cohort study in Sweden of individuals born preterm and/or small for gestational age between 1925 and 1949 (n=3364), showed a 7 fold increase in risk of oesophageal adenocarcinoma in the cohort compared with a control group born after 35 weeks of gestation having a birthweight of ›2000g. (RR 7.27, 95% CI 1.98, 18.62). Those with a birthweight ‹2000g regardless of gestation were at greatest risk (RR 11.5, 95% CI 1.39, 41.5) [Kaijser *et al.*, 2005], though there were few cases. It was postulated that the increased prevalence of infantile gastro-oesophageal reflux in preterm infants may be an explanation.

301. A subsequent population-based nested case-control study in Sweden (67 cases of oesophageal adenocarcinoma; 93 cases of cardia adenocarcinoma; 474 controls) found that birthweight was not associated with risk of any of the studied cancers, although gestational age at birth was negatively associated with risk of adenocarcinoma [Akre *et al.*, 2006].

302. There is insufficient evidence to support an association between birthweight and oesophageal or gastric cancers.

4.5.6 All cancer risk

4.5.6.1 Birthweight, size and body composition at birth and all cancer risk

303. A prospective study of 1,080 Swedish women observed a statistically significant positive association between birthweight and length and all cancers [Andersson *et al.*, 2001]. When risks for combined hormone-related cancers (104 cases) or breast cancer alone (62 cases) were analysed separately, the association with birthweight was not statistically significant. There was a doubling in risk of non-hormonal cancers (158 cases) at the highest quintile of birthweight compared to the lowest quintile (RR 2.07, 95% CI 1.22, 3.5; P_{trend} = 0.003).

304. Another prospective Swedish study of 11,166 subjects (2,685 primary cancers during 41 years follow-up) observed an 8% increased risk of overall cancer incidence per standard deviation increase in birthweight for gestational age for men of any age (RR 1.08, 95% CI 1.02, 1.14). Amongst women, risk was confined to those less than 50 years old and the effect was mainly attributable to premenopausal breast cancer [McCormack *et al.*, 2005].

305. A prospective study of 13,830 people in Finland investigated the relationship between size and weight at birth and all-cause adult mortality [Kajantie *et al.*,

2005]. The effects of weight, length and ponderal index at birth on cancer and cardiovascular disease were examined separately. Lower birthweight and shorter birth length were associated with increased all-cause mortality in females (P_{trend} = 0.01 and P_{trend} < 0.0001 respectively) but not in males (P_{trend} = 0.2 and P_{trend} = 0.4 respectively). When 630 cancer deaths were analysed separately, lower birthweight was associated with decreased mortality in males (P_{trend} = 0.02) but not in females (P_{trend} = 0.6). Birth length was not associated with cancer mortality risk, but ponderal index at birth was inversely associated with risk in males (P_{trend} = 0.01). When mortality from cardiovascular disease (n=654) was analysed separately, birthweight and birth length were inversely associated with mortality in both men and women but ponderal index was inversely associated with cardiovascular disease in men only. This study suggests that, in men, the acknowledged inverse association between cardiovascular disease and birthweight or size (see section 4.2.1.1) is offset by a positive association between cancer and birthweight.

4.5.6.2   Postnatal growth and all cancer risk

306.   The World Cancer Research Fund systematic review of cohort and case-control studies observed positive associations between adult height and risk of several cancers [World Cancer Research Fund / American Institute for Cancer Research, 2007]. The most consistent associations were found in relation to colorectal cancer and postmenopausal breast cancer, although associations were also reported for many other cancers too. Since adult height is particularly determined by birth size, age at puberty and the rate of appendicular skeletal growth, it seems likely that nutritional exposures in early life play some part in causation (see sections 3.1 – 3.3).

4.6   Bone mineral density and bone mass

307.   The interpretation of studies investigating the influence of early life on later bone growth is complicated because of the difficulty in distinguishing the influence of pre- and postnatal exposures from those of current body weight and size. Anthropometric measures track through childhood, and bone and body size are important determinants of bone mineral mass at all ages [Cole, 2004b].

4.6.1   Maternal diet, maternal nutritional status and offspring bone mineral density/bone mass

308.   Analysis of the Avon Longitudinal Study of Parents and Children (ALSPAC) found that maternal UVB exposure (which is important for synthesis of vitamin D in the skin) is related to bone size at age 9.9 years. A positive association was found with bone mineral content and bone mineral density, but not area-adjusted bone mineral content (measured by DXA) [Sayers & Tobias, 2009].

309.   An observational study of 198 white women and their offspring in Southampton (latitude 50°) [Javaid et al., 2006] observed that 31% of mothers had serum 25(OH) vitamin D concentrations (a marker of vitamin D status) between 27.5-50 nmol/l in late pregnancy. In 18%, serum 25(OH) vitamin D concentrations were less than 27.5 nmol/l. Whole-body bone mineral content (measured by DXA) of the

offspring at 9 years of age was greatest among children born to mothers who had higher plasma 25(OH) vitamin D concentrations in pregnancy. Both the estimated exposure to UVB radiation during late pregnancy and the maternal use of vitamin D supplements predicted maternal 25(OH) vitamin D concentrations and childhood bone mass. A low umbilical venous blood calcium concentration also predicted lower childhood bone mass (p=0.025 after adjustment for gestational age, current chronological age, and umbilical-venous albumin concentration).

310. Further analysis of the same cohort of pregnant women and their offspring at 9 years of age, observed that a high "prudent maternal diet score" (high intakes of fruit and vegetables, wholemeal bread, rice and pasta and low intakes of processed foods) was associated with greater bone size and areal bone mineral density (measured by DXA) in the offspring [Cole *et al.*, 2009]. Whole body bone mineral content was 11% greater and whole body bone area 8% greater than in children whose mothers showed a low prudent diet score.

311. A study in Pune, India observed that maternal mid-trimester intake of calcium rich foods was correlated with both total body and spinal bone mineral content and bone mineral density (measured by DXA) in the offspring at six years of age. Median calcium intake in this population of women was low (about 280 mg/d) and vitamin D status was not documented [Ganpule *et al.*, 2006]. However, another study of well nourished British women investigating changes in bone mineral status and size during pregnancy, found that calcium intake (including supplements) before and during pregnancy did not affect bone mineral status (measured by DXA) [Olausson *et al.*, 2008].

312. Furthermore, in a placebo controlled randomised trial conducted in The Gambia, a maternal calcium supplement of 1500 mg calcium per day given between 20 weeks gestation and delivery had no effect on maternal breastmilk calcium concentration or infant bone mineral status (measured using single photon absorptiometry of the radius and whole body DXA). Mean calcium intake in the control group was 360 mg calcium per day [Jarjou *et al.*, 2006].

313. In the Avon Longitudinal Study of Parents and Children (ALSPAC) maternal intakes of potassium, magnesium and folate measured using a food frequency questionnaire at 32 weeks of gestation were correlated with bone mineral content measured by DXA at the age of 9 years. Potassium intake was positively correlated with total body bone mineral content and magnesium and folate intake with spinal bone mineral content [Tobias *et al.*, 2005].

4.6.2 Birthweight and offspring bone mineral density/bone mass

314. Several studies have reported a weak positive association between adult bone mass, skeletal size and birthweight [Cooper *et al.*, 2005].

4.6.3 Postnatal growth and offspring bone mineral density/bone mass

315. A Finnish cohort comprising 7,086 men and women [Cooper *et al.*, 2001] identified two risk factors for hip fracture risk after adjustment for age and sex: tall maternal

height (p<0.001) and a low rate of childhood growth (height, p=0.006; weight, p=0.01). The ratio was 1.9 (95% CI 1.1, 3.2) among those whose rate of childhood height gain was below the lowest quartile for the cohort, compared with those above the highest quartile. Sex differences were also observed in patterns of growth that predicted future hip fracture. Among those later sustaining fractures, boys had a constant deficit in height and weight between ages 7 and 15 years, and girls had an increasing deficit in weight but delayed height gain.

4.6.4 Early feeding and offspring bone mineral density/bone mass

316. No association has been found between duration of breastfeeding or adherence to current guidelines on infant feeding, and bone mass in early childhood at 4 years [Harvey et al., 2009].

4.7 Summary of epidemiological evidence

317. The majority of studies looking at the relationship between birthweight and CHD risk show modest inverse associations: studies of CVD risk factors (blood pressure, serum cholesterol) and birthweight also suggest small inverse associations (section 4.2). Taken together, lower birthweight, lower weight at one year, and increased BMI in childhood are associated with an increased risk of CVD.

318. Lower birthweight is associated with increased risk of subsequent type 2 diabetes in most populations [Whincup et al., 2008] although there may be some increase in risk at the upper end of the birthweight distribution as well (section 4.4.1). Increase in BMI after the age of 2 and early adiposity rebound increases the risk of type 2 diabetes in adult life, although this association is weak when adjusted for other variables (see section 4.4.2).

319. There is inconsistent evidence that breastfeeding influences subsequent cardiovascular mortality (section 4.2.1.3) although infants who are not breastfed tend to have slightly higher blood pressure and serum total cholesterol concentrations in adult life (sections 4.2.2.3 and 4.2.3.2). Infants who are not breastfed are also at greater risk of type 2 diabetes (section 4.4.3) and are more likely to be obese (as defined by BMI) in later life (section 4.3.3).

320. Higher birthweight is associated with higher BMI in later life though there remains some doubt about what BMI reflects in this context. The few studies of body composition that have been able to resolve separately the fat and lean mass components, suggest that high birthweight may be associated with relatively greater lean mass, whereas low birthweight is associated with relatively greater fat mass (section 4.3).

321. Greater birthweight and birth size are associated with an increase in risk of certain cancers in later life, notably childhood leukaemia (section 4.5.1.2) and breast cancer (particularly in premenopausal women) (section 4.5.2.1). Taller height during childhood and adolescence and more rapid height gain are also associated with an increased risk of premenopausal breast cancer (section 4.5.2.2). However, greater

body fatness during childhood and adolescence is associated with a reduced risk of breast cancer, particularly premenopausal breast cancer (section 4.5.2.2).

322. Higher maternal UVB exposure and circulating 25(OH) vitamin D concentrations are associated with greater offspring bone size in later childhood, but the relationship with maternal calcium intake or the effects of maternal calcium supplementation are not clear (section 4.6.1). A low rate of childhood growth (i.e. height and weight) may also be a risk factor for later hip fracture (section 4.6.3).

5　Putative Mechanisms and their Implications

323.　Epidemiology indicates association between many aspects of early life nutrition and later chronic disease, but the strength and magnitude of these effects are modest and sometimes inconsistent. As indicated earlier (section 4.1), epidemiology helps to frame research questions, and design empirical approaches to establish causality and examine possible mechanisms.

324.　The complexity of diet and changes in eating behaviour during the lifecourse present difficulties when speculating upon the role of particular nutrients. Diet is a set of variables: nutrients, non-nutritional components, single foods, food groups and the physical characteristics of foods could all be considered exposures. Across populations and groups of people, the differential effects of stressors on nutrient metabolism may require additional consideration; for example, the effect of calcium supplementation during pregnancy on blood pressure in the offspring was strongest in those whose body mass index lay in the top quartile [Belizan et al., 1997]. Similarly a higher BMI in adulthood was more strongly associated with CHD risk among women who were small at birth than among those who were not [Rich-Edwards et al., 2005].

325.　Ideally, human intervention studies are needed to explore mechanisms, though pragmatic and ethical factors may constrain recruitment of subjects to specific population groups. For example, the early feeding studies outlined in the next section mainly involve preterm infants. Findings from such studies cannot be generalised to the whole population, though lessons may be learned.

326.　There is additional information from studies where risk markers for chronic disease are measured in individuals whose mothers took part in RCTs of nutritional interventions during pregnancy (predominantly protein/energy supplementation and some micronutrient supplementation) [Stein et al., 2006; Hoddinot et al., 2008; Kinra et al., 2008; Hawkesworth et al., 2008; Vaidya et al., 2008; Hawkesworth et al., 2009; Stewart et al., 2009]. However, these studies are not considered because they are based on populations from developing countries in whom there is a high prevalence of chronic energy or micronutrient restriction, and again it is difficult to extrapolate the data and apply it to the UK population.

327.　Human studies examine predominantly postnatal effects and we remain largely dependent on animal evidence to inform us about mechanisms which operate during pregnancy. Consideration of animal studies follows in section 5.2.

5.1　Human intervention studies

328.　Randomised controlled feeding studies have been conducted in British preterm infants weighing under 1850g at birth [Singhal & Lucas, 2004]. Infants were recruited to two parallel trials conducted in the 1980s. In one, they were randomly allocated to receive either breastmilk donated by unrelated lactating women or a nutrient-enriched "preterm formula". In the other, they received either the same "preterm formula" or standard "term formula". In both trials, infants were sub-divided into groups according to whether mothers provided their own breastmilk or not.

329. Significantly faster early weight gain, linear and head circumference growth was seen among those randomised to nutrient-enriched "preterm formula" rather than banked breastmilk, which was particularly low in energy density [Singhal & Lucas, 2004]. However, at school age (mean 7.5 years) no between-group differences were apparent in weight or any measures of size, including BMI and skinfold thickness [Morley & Lucas, 2000].

330. Follow-up of some of these children at 13-16 years of age indicated that mean and diastolic arterial blood pressure were significantly greater amongst those randomly allocated to formula as opposed to banked breast milk [Singhal et al., 2001]. In separate analyses, the ratio of LDL to HDL cholesterol was significantly lower in adolescents randomised to banked breastmilk compared with preterm formula [Singhal et al., 2004], as was fasting plasma insulin [Singhal et al., 2003]. The ratio of leptin to fat mass in adolescence was also higher in those who were randomised to breastmilk or standard formula as opposed to nutrient-dense preterm formula. It was suggested that the programming of relative leptin concentrations by early diet could be one mechanism that links early nutrition with later obesity.

331. In the Republic of Belarus, a cluster-randomised trial was undertaken to evaluate the effect of the UNICEF Baby Friendly Hospital Initiative on breastfeeding and disease outcomes. Altogether, 17,046 term baby-mother pairs were recruited and followed up through the early years of life. Infants born in the intervention group gained in weight and length more quickly in the first few months than those born in the control hospitals [Kramer et al., 2002]. This contrasts with observational analysis of the trial data (mentioned earlier in section 3.5.2; Kramer et al., 2004). Later analysis of infants followed to 6.5 years of age revealed no difference in physical parameters or blood pressure between those born in intervention or control hospitals [Kramer et al., 2007] (see section 3.5.2).

332. The effect of infant protein intake on growth has been studied by randomly assigning formula-fed infants to receive infant and follow-on formulas differing in protein concentration. Those with higher protein intake had higher weight, but not greater length, at 2 years of age [Koletzko et al., 2009b]. It was suggested that a higher intake of protein from infant formula might stimulate secretion of IGF-1 and consequently cell proliferation leading to increased adipose tissue mass [Koletzko et al., 2009a].

333. In an American trial white infants were randomly allocated to receive solid foods from 3 or 6 months of age. No differences were found in growth rate or body composition (measured by DXA) at 12 months [Mehta et al., 1998].

334. An RCT examined the effect of dietary sodium on the blood pressure of 476 full-term new born infants assigned to a low sodium diet (0.1g/4.8 mmol per day) or

a diet providing 0.3g/13.4 mmol per day during the first 6 months of life ("diet" included formula and solid foods) [Hofman et al., 1983]. At 6 months, a significant difference was observed in systolic blood pressure between the two groups, which was on average 2.1 mmHg lower in infants fed the low sodium diet compared to infants on the higher sodium diet. One hundred and sixty-seven of these children were re-examined fifteen years later: adjusted systolic blood pressure remained 3.6 mmHg lower (95% CI −6.6, −0.5) and diastolic pressure 2.2 mmHg lower (95% CI −4.5, 0.2) in those assigned during infancy to the low sodium group (n=71) [Geleijnse et al., 1997].

5.2 Animal intervention studies and epigenetics

335. Experimental interventions utilising animal models have enabled more direct evaluation of the effects of maternal nutrient exposure (usually nutrient restriction) upon offspring size, body composition and metabolic competence. Collectively, the results support the implications of the human epidemiological studies described above: they demonstrate that the timing, degree and duration of nutritional restriction operate independently to determine the risk of chronic disease in later life [Lucas, 1991; Seckl, 1998; Rasmussen, 2001]. Importantly, animal studies have also identified how modification of the epigenome through nutritional exposure might explain "programming" phenomena [Gallou-Kabani & Junien 2005; Liu et al., 2008; Gluckman et al., 2009].

336. Dietary restriction during early pregnancy in rats, particularly around the time of conception, influences placentation to result in a relatively high placental/offspring body weight ratio at term [Langley-Evans, 2001]. Similar effects have been seen in pregnant rats fed an iron deficient diet [Crowe et al., 1995; Gambling et al., 2003]. Studies in sheep show that the outcomes depend on the timing of dietary restriction during pregnancy [Godfrey, 1998]: restriction between the time of conception and mid-gestation results in a large placenta with a normal weight fetus [Symonds et al., 2000]. Conversely, when ewes are fed adequately at conception and are then given higher nutrient intakes, there is a reduction in relative placental weight [Robinson et al., 1994; Godfrey, 1998].

337. Reducing the intake of a variety of macronutrients (e.g. protein) and micronutrients (e.g. iron, zinc, calcium) during pregnancy, particularly during late gestation, can reduce birthweight and predispose the offspring to hypertension and the development of diabetes in later life [Crowe et al., 1995; Bertram & Hanson, 2001; Ozanne & Hales, 2002; Gambling et al., 2003; Tomat et al., 2008]. The fact that restriction of several nutrients can independently produce similar phenotypic outcomes [Harding, 2005] suggests that it is the disruption of development itself, rather than any specific nutrient deficiency, which induces these clinical features. It is important to recognise that nutrient and energy restrictions within the normal range of dietary experience are sufficient to effect phenotypic change in animal studies.

338. Moreover, reduction in birthweight is not a pre-requisite for increased susceptibility to increased blood pressure or altered substrate metabolism. Dietary manipulations such as those described above have been associated in pregnant rats with marked

post-weaning changes in the offspring's blood pressure and glucose tolerance without any change in birthweight [Dahri et al., 1991; Langley & Jackson, 1994; Langley et al., 1994; Desai et al., 1995]. Similarly, rat pups from dams fed protein-restricted diets had fewer nephrons in their kidneys [Marchand & Langley-Evans, 2001], although the weight of the kidneys was no different to that of offspring whose mothers were fed adequately.

339.   Central obesity, another key element of the metabolic syndrome, has also been related to nutrient exposure in early life [Remacle et al., 2004]; redistribution of fat deposition in the rat pups of protein-restricted dams was also accompanied by an appetite preference for high-fat foods [Bellinger et al., 2004]. Again, nutrient imbalance appears to be the triggering event [Langley-Evans, 2001].

340.   Thus animal models have demonstrated clear relationships between maternal dietary manipulation during gestation and the later appearance of features of metabolic syndrome in their offspring. These experimental findings are consistent with associations observed in humans. The mechanisms that could explain these findings include: disruption of organ development, disruption of the endocrine environment and epigenetics. These are not mutually exclusive.

341.   *Disruption of organ development.* Organs and tissues develop from a set of progenitor (stem) cells and tissue development follows a strictly ordered pattern. Anything that disrupts this pattern can have significant consequences [Brameld et al., 1998]. If the nutritional insult occurs during the differentiation phase of an organ, then the organ would be expected to be of normal size, but with an altered tissue architecture. Stress in the proliferative phase would result in a normal tissue architecture, but reduced number of cells. This "remodelling" has been studied most comprehensively in the kidney. Exposing rats to a low protein diet can result in a decrease of up to 40% in the number of nephrons [Langley-Evans et al., 1999; Vehaskari et al., 2001], an effect which seems to be constant across models and species [Lisle et al., 2003; Gilbert et al., 2005; Hoppe et al., 2007; Tomat et al., 2008]. Interestingly, reduction in nephron number is also associated with hypertension in humans, suggesting the animal data may explain some of the aspects of fetal programming in humans.

342.   Other tissues that show evidence of remodelling include placenta [Lewis et al., 2001; Gambling et al., 2004], brain [Bennis-Taleb et al., 1999] and pancreas: maternal protein restriction reduces the number of functional B cells in the offspring by half [Snoeck et al., 1990].

343.   *Disruption of the endocrine environment.* Endocrine changes during pregnancy can not only alter cellular responses, but may also change homeostatic regulation. Of particular interest is the effect of early nutritional stress on the hypothalamic-pituitary-adrenal axis and steroid hormonal influences.

344.   Alteration of glucocorticoid metabolism by a variety of early life stresses could produce a relatively limited, but common, range of later programmed responses [Langley-Evans, 2006]. Effects on the offspring can include reduced birthweight, hyperglycemia, hypertension and reduced nephron number (as described earlier

in this section). Pharmacological blockade of maternal glucocorticoid synthesis prevents the programming of hypertension in the offspring of the pregnant rats fed protein-restricted diets [Langley-Evans, 2001].

345. There is a large glucorticoid concentration gradient across the placenta, with maternal circulating concentrations 100-1000 times greater than those in the fetal circulation. This arises in part from the degradation, by placental enzyme 11β-hydroxysteroid dehydrogenase type 2, of corticosteroids such as cortisol to less active forms (e.g. cortisone). This may be a means of protecting the fetus from maternal glucocorticoid activity [Seckl & Meaney, 2004]. Additionally, the breakdown of maternal glucocorticoids also ensures the integrity and independence of the fetal hypothalamo-pituitary-adrenal axis [Edwards et al., 1993].

346. Pregnant rats fed protein restricted diets show reduced placental activity and expression of 11β-hydroxysteroid dehydrogenase type 2 [Langley-Evans et al., 1996; Bertram et al., 2001], thus exposing the conceptus to greater amounts of maternal glucocorticoid. Simultaneously there may be increased expression of glucocorticoid receptors in the fetal kidney, liver, lung, and brain [Bertram et al., 2001]. The latter may be an independent feature, a result of the raised glucocorticoid levels [Freeman et al., 2004], or a combination of both. Either way, increased glucocorticoid sensitivity arises as the consequence of nutritional deprivation during pregnancy. Increased expression of glucocorticoid receptors has also been observed in the lungs, livers, adrenal glands and kidneys of lambs from ewes fed restricted diets during pregnancy [Whorwood et al., 2001; Brennan et al., 2005; Gnanalingham et al., 2005].

347. Restricting maternal protein intake in rats during pregnancy, lactation, or both, also alters the expression of genes involved in lipid metabolism. Expression of the enzymes acetyl-CoA carboxylase and fatty acid synthase were increased in the liver of rat offspring fed a protein-restricted diet during pregnancy and lactation [Maloney et al., 2003]. Additionally the offspring of rats fed a protein-restricted diet during pregnancy showed increased blood triacylglycerol and non-esterified fatty acid concentrations [Burdge et al., 2004], raised expression of hepatic peroxisomal proliferator-activated receptor-α (PPARα) (which regulates fatty acid clearance pathways), and up-regulation of acyl-CoA oxidase [Burdge et al., 2004; Lillycrop et al., 2005].

348. The effects of prenatal nutritional restriction on birthweight, glucose tolerance and the hypothalamic-pituitary axis observed in the animal's offspring, can persist for several generations despite an adequate nutritional supply in subsequent pregnancies [Drake & Walker, 2004].

349. Transgenerational effects of a protein-restricted diet during pregnancy have been demonstrated in the rat model. Insulin resistance has been noted in two subsequent generations (F_1 and F_2 generations) of dams (F_0) who were nutritionally deprived, although the F_1 had been fed adequately throughout their maturation and pregnancy. Subsequently, defective homeostasis of glucose has been shown to extend even through the F_1 and F_2 to the F_3 generations [Benyshek et al., 2006].

350.   These data illustrate that the mechanisms underlying phenotypic change alter cell types and numbers, tissue remodelling (through influences on apoptosis), glucocorticoid levels and receptor levels, and lipid metabolism. The changes described in animals reflect events occurring at various stages between the pre-implantation and neonatal periods, and it appears that diverse stimuli can induce similar functional and structural outcomes. Several explanations for these observations have been posited. These include effects of a common gene or gene pathway (the "gatekeeper" hypothesis), and a possible role for epigenetic phenomena [Gallou-Kabani & Junien 2005; Liu *et al.*, 2008; Gluckman *et al.*, 2009].

351.   *"Epigenetics"* describes the cellular mechanisms stabilising processes by which inherited genetic information in the chromosomes (i.e. the genome) is transcribed. The term literally means "on top of genes" and it refers to the superimposed regulation of gene expression. By controlling which of the 30,000 or so genes in the human genome are functioning, epigenetic influences determine the functional and architectural development of cells, tissues and organs. Such a mechanism would be capable of mediating the organism's response to external stimuli such as qualitative and quantitative nutritional supply, stress and environmental chemicals [Liu *et al.*, 2008; Weaver, 2009]. Epigenetics embraces the understanding of how regulatory elements "switch" genes "on or off", and how this is synchronised spatially and temporally.

352.   Epigenetic marking brought about by exposure to external stimuli during development differs from the phenomenon of genomic imprinting, the epigenetic marking of parental origin at certain chromosomal domains. Imprinted genes may have central roles in controlling fetal demand for, and placental supply of, maternal nutrients. Inheritance of specific transcripts of imprinted genes, such as the placenta-specific IGF-2 transcript in rodents, could control the placental supply of nutrients irrespective of maternal nutritional state. Knockout mouse models[xxx] have shown such effects on placental transport capacity, consistent with the role of IGF-2 in modulating placental supply and fetal demand for nutrients [Reik *et al.*, 2003].

353.   It is noteworthy that mechanisms and regulatory controls involved in epigenetics may operate intermittently or continuously, for a short or a prolonged period. They may persist through mitotic division to survive in cell lines from early life to adulthood or may pass into the gamete (germ cells) through meiosis, and thus operate transgenerationally. Thus, subsequent generations inherit not only a genetic blueprint (genome), but also a heritable element of control (the epigenome) over its expression. The epigenome is, however, variable; characterising better how it is controlled and sustained is one aim of animal experimentation intended to explore mechanisms suggested by human epidemiological studies.

354.   Gluckman and colleagues (2009) have reviewed recently current understanding of the epigenetic mechanisms underpinning metabolic and cardiovascular diseases. They demonstrate how the three components, genome, development,

---

xxx A genetically engineered mouse in which one or more existing genes have been replaced or disrupted through a targeted mutation.

and environment, interact to determine an organism's growth, metabolism and potential susceptibility to disease in later life. These predetermining interactions affect gametogenesis, conception, histogenesis, organogenesis, and early life adaptation to changes in substrate metabolism. Risk of disease is thought to increase when there is a mismatch between relative nutrient supply between the pre and postnatal environment.

355.   The molecular processes affecting epigenetic control include methylation by DNA methyl transferase of cytosine-guanine (CpG) islands[xxxi] in the 5' promoter regions of the DNA in genes. Methylation of CpG islands silences gene expression. Gene-specific methylation can be maintained through mitosis [Bird, 2002]. Another mechanism is chromatin modification through histone acetylation [Surani, 2001]. This process controls the physical condensation of the chromatin wound around a histone: condensed or tightly wound chromatin is in a silent state because the responsive elements and regulators are denied access to gene promoter sequences. An extensive number of histone and chromatin modifications have now been recognised but the interaction, stability, and control of these have not been fully characterised [Liu et al., 2008].

356.   Epigenetic modification of gene expression has the potential to explain how maternal nutritional status influences fetal phenotype [Burdge et al., 2007a]. In the context of the phenomena described here DNA methylation is the most extensively used marker of epigenetic influence.

357.   Methylation of promoter regions may be induced during the early development of the embryo or during the differentiation of individual tissues [Bird, 2002] which is accompanied by a progressive decrease in the methylation of specific genes [Grainger et al., 1983; Benvenisty et al., 1985]. This variation in the timing and direction of methylation events suggests a mechanism by which the timing of a nutritional stimulus determines phenotypic outcomes.

358.   DNA methylation requires the dietary supply of nutrients involved in the methylation cycle. Several vitamins including folate, riboflavin, vitamin B_6, and vitamin B_{12} each act as cofactors for the enzyme steps of methylation. They are specifically involved in the synthesis of S-adenosylmethionine, the primary methyl group donor for DNA methylation. Controlled studies in the pregnant agouti mouse have shown that varying the dietary intake of methyl donors such as choline and betaine alters offspring coat colour through increased methylation of seven CpG islands in the promoter region of the agouti gene[xxxii] [Wolff et al., 1998; Cooney et al., 2002; Waterland & Jirtle, 2003].

xxxi A 200-bp stretch of DNA with a C+G content of 50% and an observed CpG/expected CpG ratio in excess of 0.6. CpG islands are useful markers for genes in organisms containing 5-methylcytosine in their genomes. In addition, CpG islands located in the promoter regions of genes can play important roles in gene silencing during processes such as X-chromosome inactivation, imprinting, and silencing of intragenomic parasites [Takai & Jones, 2002].

xxxii Agouti gene is expressed in the hair follicle and promotes yellow hair colour as an antagonist to the activity of the alpha-melanocyte stimulating hormone (α-MSH) on the melanocortin receptor (MCR). The ectopic expression of the agouti protein in regions of the brain that are responsible for the body weight homeostasis results in hyperphagia and subsequently in obesity [Stutz et al., 2005].

359. Methylation patterns are largely established during embryogenesis or in early development: demethylation (or erasure) of the genome of the embryo occurs just after conception and remethylation occurs before implantation [Reik et al., 2001]. DNA methylation plays a key role in cell differentiation by silencing the expression of specific genes during the development and differentiation of individual tissues. Some genes appear to show gradations of promoter demethylation associated with developmental changes in role of the gene product [Burdge et al., 2007a].

360. There are several tiers to epigenetic mechanisms, which when integrated, may lead to adaptive effects [Liu et al., 2008; Gluckman et al., 2009]. In pregnant rats fed protein-restricted diets, there is a decrease in methylation and an increase in the expression of PPAR-α and glucocorticoid receptor genes in the liver and heart of the offspring after weaning [Lillycrop et al., 2005]. Hypomethylation of the glucocorticoid receptor gene is associated with several modifications of the histone associated with the promoter for the glucocorticoid receptor gene which facilitate its transcription [Lillycrop et al., 2007].

361. The existence of epigenetic differential control was illustrated by feeding a protein-restricted diet to rats during pregnancy. This induced a reduction in DNA methyltransferase 1 expression and binding of the enzyme at the glucocorticoid receptor promoter [Lillycrop et al., 2007]. However, there was no reduction in the expression of other DNA methyltransferases [Lillycrop et al., 2007]. This suggested that hypomethylation of the glucocorticoid receptor promoter was induced by a reduced capacity to maintain patterns of cytosine methylation during mitosis rather than active demethylation or a de novo failure of methylation.

362. Effects of altered methylation status may be deduced from observations that the induction of hypertension and endothelial dysfunction in the offspring of rats fed a protein-restricted diet during pregnancy could be prevented by supplementing the diet with glycine or folic acid [Jackson et al., 2002; Brawley et al., 2004]. Similarly, hypomethylation of the hepatic glucocorticoid and PPARα promoters was prevented by a 5-fold increase in the folic acid content of a protein-restricted diet [Lillycrop et al., 2005], resulting in an increase in glucocorticoid and PPARα expression.

363. Pregnant rats fed a protein-restricted diet showed increased plasma homocysteine concentration in early gestation [Petrie et al., 2002]. DNA methyltransferase expression is reduced by homocysteine and increased by folic acid. Lower DNA methyltransferase 1 (Dnmt1) expression induced by the protein-restricted diet was prevented by increasing the folic acid content of the protein-restricted diet [Lillycrop et al., 2007] and is consistent with a role for Dnmt1 in the induction of an altered phenotype [Jackson et al., 2002; Brawley et al., 2004]. This is consistent with the hypothesis that alteration of 1-carbon unit metabolism through maternal dietary manipulation affects epigenetic regulation through alteration of DNA methylation at promoter sites.

364. When the female offspring of rats fed a protein-restricted diet during pregnancy were mated and fed an unrestricted diet throughout pregnancy and lactation, the

80 day old F_2 males had comparably low degrees of methylation of their hepatic glucocorticoid and PPARα promoters as had the 80 day old male F_1 generation [Burdge et al., 2007b]. This is consistent with other evidence of inter-generational transmission of phenotype and of part of the epigenome [Burdge et al., 2007a].

365. The role of epigenetics in human disease is becoming better appreciated. Altered methylation of DNA [Szyf et al., 2004] and altered methylation/acetylation of the histones associated with DNA [Fraga et al., 2005] has been noted in human cancers. Altered DNA methylation has also been associated with atherosclerosis in humans [Castro et al., 2003] and similar patterns of altered global DNA methylation have been observed in mouse and rabbit atherosclerotic lesions [Hiltunen et al., 2002]. Studies in an atherogenic mouse model have shown that altered DNA methylation precedes the development of atherosclerosis [Lund et al., 2004]. Furthermore, proliferation of vascular smooth muscle cells may be influenced by changes in DNA methylation [Post et al., 1999; Ying et al., 2000]. DNA methylation has also been shown to vary with alcohol exposure in humans [Bonsch et al., 2004; Bonsch et al., 2005].

366. Clearly, knowledge about epigenetic regulation of genetic expression and development in animal models and in the context of human development and later disease is incomplete. As yet, there is no indication in humans of a dose-response relationship for epigenetic associations, though it is noteworthy that alteration of phenotype in animals can be induced by nutrient and energy restrictions within the normal range of dietary exposures. It should be appreciated that any of the nutritional manipulations applied in animal experiments may imbalance the diet in other respects, for example, in relation to micronutrient intake or requirements. Many mechanisms involved in regulating gene expression have been identified, but the precise means whereby these are initiated by environmental, nutritional and behavioural stimuli is currently unknown. For example it is not clear why dietary manipulation modifies the expression of one gene or gene family but not another. Nor is it understood why, or indeed whether, changes in the epigenetic marking in one cell type are matched in all. Collectively, these limitations and uncertainties make it difficult at the moment to apply knowledge of human epigenetics to public health nutritional strategies and interventions, but they signal the need for concern.

5.2.1   Limitations of animal experimental models

367. Animal studies allow controlled nutritional interventions that would not be feasible or ethical in humans (see section 2.2). Although they offer insight into mechanisms that may explain the epidemiological data, they have limitations. These include species differences, use of animals less mature at birth than humans, use of inbred strains, small group sizes and stressors not clearly relevant to human experience [Hartung, 2008; McMullen & Mostyn, 2009; Symonds & Burdge, 2009; Symonds et al., 2009].

368. Animal models nevertheless allow identification of precise developmental windows in which early nutrition can contribute to later disease. Thus, data from both epidemiological and animal research complement one another.

5.3 Summary

369. The epidemiological evidence in the previous chapter shows that a number of early life markers of nutritional status are correlated with long-term disease risk. In particular birthweight and birth size, early feeding, and the rate of growth in early life modify the prevalence of cardiovascular disease and its risk factors (such as blood pressure, adiposity and glucose tolerance) and certain cancers.

370. Human studies provide some insight into the mechanisms related to pre and postnatal effects on development of disease in adulthood, but so far, only animal evidence can provide an understanding about prenatal events that might programme risk for later life.

371. Controlled studies in animals have yielded insight into the mechanisms that underlie epidemiologically observed associations between human markers of fetal nutrient and energy restriction and adult disease outcome.

372. Specific epidemiological evidence from populations affected by severe food shortage during gestation or early life implies that the timing of nutritional restriction in humans may predict the structural and functional effects observed in the offspring's adult life. These situations have imposed severe generalised macronutrient and micronutrient restriction. There is little human evidence linking long term outcome to the effect of restricting intake of specific nutrients in fetal or early postnatal life.

373. Similarly, experimental dietary restriction in pregnant animals has shown that the timing, degree and duration of nutrient and energy restriction exert a stronger influence on fetal development than the specific nature of nutrient restriction. Limitation of micronutrient or macronutrient intake sufficient to achieve dietary imbalance may alter phenotype through disruption of the normal sequence of tissue development.

374. The consequence of this process is alteration of the offspring phenotype, which may be evident as change in body weight, size, body composition or function. Each may be altered independently, though there are well described correlations between alteration of function, of organ architecture and of tissue composition.

375. Understanding of the processes by which nutrients may alter gene expression suggests mechanisms by which nutrient supply to the fetus may induce change in phenotype at the cellular and tissue level. Of particular interest is the observation that imbalance in the supply of those nutrients involved in the methylation cycle may induce change in observable characteristics.

376. Several mechanisms which are not mutually exclusive may induce fetal programming. The endocrinological balance of the mother and feto-placental unit may be altered by changes in the expression of placental 11β-hydroxysteroid dehydrogenase and of fetal glucocortcoid receptors. Additionally, alterations in the rate of cell division during the stages of proliferation or differentiation may result in changed organ size or tissue architecture. Such changes may offer an explanation for the

observed relationship between impairment of fetal development and physical or emotional stresses imposed on the pregnant mother.

377.   Epigenetic effects have been invoked to explain the inter-generational effects of nutrient restriction observed in pregnant animals. It is possible that they may explain inter-generational effects observed in the offspring born to women exposed to famine during fetal life.

6 Implications for Maternal and Child Nutrition in the UK

378. Epidemiological and experimental evidence suggests that it is important to provide adequate nutrient supply early in development and ensure it is maintained throughout the reproductive continuum from embryonic or fetal life to pregnancy and lactation.

379. In the following sections, implications for public health identified in previous chapters are placed in a UK context. The chapter first examines current UK trends in birthweight, infant feeding practices and the diet and nutrition of young children in the UK. The nutritional status of women of childbearing age in the UK is then reviewed, and information from local studies of pregnant women collated. Finally, population trends in BMI are reviewed, particularly in relation to pregnancy outcome. National data are cited wherever possible.

6.1 Current trends in birthweight

380. Although birthweight is not a sensitive descriptor of variations in fetal nutritional experience (see section 3.2.3) it remains a marker for chronic disease risk. As described earlier (see section 3.2) birthweight marks a process, which is related to later disease risk, but the exact relationship is not linear and is complex. Extremes of birthweight may carry additional specific risks.

381. It is noteworthy that the mean birthweight of babies born in the UK to women of Caribbean, sub-Saharan African, and South Asian (Indian) origin is lower than that of babies born to women of White European origin [Office for National Statistics, 2000].

382. A British Cohort study using nationally representative UK birthweight data found no evidence of an increase across the generations. Among mothers of Black Caribbean, Black African, Indian, Pakistani and Bangladeshi ethnicity, mean birthweights of infants born to migrant mothers were similar to those of infants whose mothers were born in the UK, although this was not adjusted for maternal height [Harding et al., 2004]. A smaller study of women of South Asian origin living in Southampton observed no increase in either maternal height or birthweight across generations [Margetts et al., 2002].

383. A study looking at birthweight and ponderal index in black and minority ethnic groups demonstrates the importance of adjusting birthweight for other variables when making comparisons across different ethnic populations [Condie, 1982]. In this study, conducted in the West Midlands, infants of South Asian origin had lower birthweight than those of African-Caribbean origin. After adjustment for maternal height, weight, parity, gestational age and fetal sex, the "corrected" birthweight of the African-Caribbean infants was lower than that of both the Indian and European

groups. The proportion of African-Caribbean infants with ponderal index <10th percentile was however lower than that of the European and Indian groups. This was interpreted as showing that African Caribbean infants were constitutionally smaller and "healthier", despite being of lower birthweight.

384. Results from the nationally representative UK Millennium Cohort Study have shown Indian, Pakistani and Bangladeshi infants to be 280g–350g lighter, and 2.5 times more likely to have low birthweight compared with White infants. Black Caribbean infants were 150g and Black African infants 70g lighter than White infants; infants in these ethnic groups were also 1.6 times more likely to be of low birthweight [Kelly et al., 2008].

385. The reasons for this ethnic variation in birthweight, and differences in birth phenotype between ethnic groups, for example with respect to body proportions at birth and maternal characteristics, are unclear. Socioeconomic factors may be important. There are also likely to be genetic influences on birthweight, but these have not been well-characterised.

6.2 Infant nutrition

386. The following section considers the impact of current infant feeding practices on later life.

6.2.1 Infant feeding practices in the UK

387. In common with the World Health Organisation, UK Health Departments recommend that babies are breastfed exclusively for the first half of infancy. Solids should be introduced at around six months when the baby is developmentally ready, and breastfeeding continued alongside increasing amounts of other foods appropriate to the diversifying diet [Department of Health, 2003].

388. In 2008, SACN reviewed the key findings from the 2005 Infant Feeding Survey [Scientific Advisory Committee on Nutrition, 2008a]. The survey showed that breastfeeding initiation and prevalence rates are increasing across the UK, although the proportion of mothers exclusively breastfeeding is relatively low at different points after birth (21% at six weeks and less than 1% at six months).

389. Solid foods were introduced later than reported in earlier quinquennial surveys; 51% of mothers introduced them by 4 months compared to 85% in 2000. In 2005, only 2% had delayed the introduction of solids until six months [Scientific Advisory Committee on Nutrition, 2008a].

390. Inequalities exist across a range of infant feeding issues and there is a consistent association with sociodemographic and educational characteristics of the mother. Young mothers and mothers from lower socioeconomic groups appear to be the least likely to adopt the infant feeding practices recommended by Health Departments [Bolling et al., 2007]. This has been highlighted by SACN and the National Institute for Health and Clinical Excellence (NICE) [Scientific Advisory Committee on Nutrition, 2008a; National Institute for Health and Clinical Excellence, 2008a].

6.2.2 Breastfeeding and long-term health outcomes

391. An extensive body of scientific evidence supports the consensus that not breastfeeding increases the risk of illness in both mothers and infants, particularly diarrhoeal disease and respiratory infection [Howie et al., 1990; Pisacane et al., 1992; Kramer & Kakuma, 2002; Ip et al., 2007; Quigley et al., 2007].

392. Whilst recognising the often inconsistent definitions used in the scientific literature about the impact of early feeding (see section 4.1.1), the epidemiological evidence considered in the previous chapters suggests that some feeding patterns are associated with health risk in later life. Observational studies have shown that breastfeeding is associated with reduced risk of childhood obesity (section 4.3.3), and possibly lower blood pressure and serum cholesterol concentrations (sections 4.2.2.3 and 4.2.3.2) and lower risk of type 2 diabetes in adulthood (section 4.4.3). Exclusive breastfeeding particularly has been associated with lower cholesterol levels in later life (section 4.2.3.2).

393. Patterns of infant feeding in the UK are strongly determined by many demographic variables including social class, mother's educational attainment, smoking behaviour, and ethnicity. Observed relationships between infant feeding method and long-term outcome are therefore highly prone to confounding. It is nevertheless clear that exclusively breastfed babies from a wide range of backgrounds show a distinctive pattern of early weight gain different to that of babies artificially fed [Scientific Advisory Committee on Nutrition, 2007a]. There is insufficient information about the influence of these early differences on later body composition and metabolic function.

6.3 The diet and nutritional status of young children in the UK

394. SACN reviewed findings from the National Diet and Nutrition Surveys (NDNS)[xxxiii] carried out between 1992 and 2001 [Scientific Advisory Committee on Nutrition, 2008c], and assessed the adequacy of dietary intakes by comparison with Dietary Reference Values (DRVs) set by the Committee on Medical Aspects of Food and Nutrition Policy (COMA) in 1991 [Department of Health, 1991] (see Appendix 2 for details). The Low Income Diet and Nutrition Survey (LIDNS) also provides data on the dietary habits and biochemical status of the low income (materially deprived)[xxxiv] population in the UK [Nelson et al., 2007] and some of the findings from this survey are also described in Appendix 2.

395. National data show that children typically have diets high in energy dense foods, saturated fat and non-milk extrinsic sugars, but low in fibre, fruits and vegetables

---

xxxiii A new government funded National Diet and Nutrition Survey (NDNS) rolling programme has been commissioned to provide detailed information on food consumption, nutrient intakes and nutritional status of the UK population from age 1½ years upwards. Year 1 results of this survey were published in February 2010 but are not considered in this report. A single diet and nutrition survey of infants and young children (4 to 18 months) has also been commissioned by government, of which results are not yet available.

xxxiv The Low Income Diet and Nutrition Survey (LIDNS) is based on a national sample of the most materially deprived households in the UK. "Low-income" used in the sections here on, refers to this population studied in the LIDNS.

(see details in Appendix 2). Consumption of energy-dense foods has been linked with obesity [Prentice & Jebb, 2003], and the proportion of children classified as obese is rising (see section 6.5 *BMI trends, obesity and pregnancy outcome*). Data also indicate that some groups also have low intakes and/or status of iron, vitamin D and vitamin A (Appendix 2) [Scientific Advisory Committee on Nutrition, 2008c].

396. Data from the national surveys show that all age groups are meeting the dietary requirements for protein (see Appendix 2). Infants in the UK whose diets rapidly diversify and who by the age of 9 months regularly eat meat, fish, eggs or reasonable quantities of milk are unlikely to be deficient in dietary protein supply [Department of Health, 1994]. It has been suggested that high protein intake in infancy might be associated with an increased risk of obesity in later life but current data are conflicting (see sections 3.5.2 and 5.1).

397. Vitamin D is particularly important for young girls as they enter childbearing years because inadequate vitamin D status has implications for pregnancy outcome, particularly bone development in the offspring (see section 4.6).

398. Low dietary iron intakes in children (see Appendix 2) are likely to be associated with an increased risk of iron deficiency and anaemia. Iron deficiency anaemia is common in certain groups of young children. High proportions of older girls have intakes below the RNI but there is current uncertainty about the DRVs for iron intake and the interpretation of measures of iron status [Scientific Advisory Committee on Nutrition, 2010].

399. Survey data also report on additional lifestyle issues including physical activity. Health Survey for England data show that there has been little variation across years in the proportions of children (aged 2-15 years) in each of the levels of physical activity[xxxv] [Chaudhury et al., 2008]. The 2008 Health Survey for England, which focused on *Physical Activity and Fitness*, reported that a higher proportion of boys than girls aged 2-15 years met the government's recommendations for physical activity, doing at least an hour of at least moderate activity every day (32% and 24% respectively) [Aresu et al., 2009]. Children in the UK (aged 10 years) have lower levels of objectively measured physical activity compared to children of similar age elsewhere in Europe [Owen et al., 2009a]. The NDNS of children aged 4-18 years showed that of children 7-18 years, girls were less active than boys and activity levels fell as age increased [Gregory et al., 2000].

6.4   Maternal nutrition

400. Section 3.1.3 showed how the mother's body composition and metabolic competence (or capacity) at conception and throughout pregnancy conserve fetal nutrient supply under normal circumstances. Pregnancy (and breastfeeding) do not require any increase in the intake of most nutrients. This does not imply that there is no increase in metabolic demand during pregnancy, but rather that such

---

xxxv   Levels of physical activity as follows: 'Meets recommendations': active for at least 60 minutes on seven days per week, 'Some activity': active for 30-59 minutes on seven days, 'Low activity': lower level of activity than that described above.

demands can be met by normal adaptation or increased efficiency of utilisation, or from stores of the nutrient [Department of Health, 1991] (see sections 3.1.2 – 3.1.4).

401.   RNIs are set for the provision of dietary energy (during the last trimester only), protein, folate, vitamin A, vitamin D, vitamin C, and two of the B vitamins (thiamin and riboflavin) during pregnancy. Dietary supplements are required to meet these reference intakes in some cases, notably provision of folic acid for pregnant women until the 12th week and those planning a pregnancy, and vitamin D for pregnant women. In the case of multiple pregnancies, SACN has stated that there is no evidence to support the suggestion that increasing nutritional intake beyond current reference intakes improves outcome [Scientific Advisory Committee on Nutrition, 2008b].

402.   There are also increased requirements for a number of nutrients for lactation. These include RNIs set for the provision of energy (for different stages of lactation), protein, folate, vitamin A, vitamin D, vitamin C, B vitamins (thiamin, riboflavin, niacin, vitamin B_{12}) and also for a number of minerals (calcium, phosphorus, magnesium, zinc, copper and selenium) [Department of Health, 1991]. Current advice is that all of these intakes can be achieved through a varied and balanced diet, apart from vitamin D, which requires a 10 microgram daily supplement for the duration of breastfeeding in order to ensure the requirement is met.

403.   The previous section referred to the nutritional status of young children using two national datasets, the National Diet and Nutrition Surveys (NDNS) and the Low Income Diet and Nutrition Survey (LIDNS). Currently there are no national data available to describe the nutritional status of pregnant women, although additional data from these national surveys can indicate the nutritional status of women of childbearing age and their likely nutritional state at the start of pregnancy. Several published UK studies have also described the nutritional status of pregnant women with regard to particular nutrients, and these are considered together in the following sections, highlighting particular areas for public health concern.

6.4.1   The nutritional status of young women and implications for pregnancy outcome

404.   Dietary advice in the UK has consistently encouraged consumption of fruit and vegetables, starchy foods, and oily fish, whilst advising limited consumption of saturated fat, salt and added sugar. Young women are advised to comply with general healthy eating advice before and during pregnancy and postpartum.

405.   However, NDNS data show that the diet and nutritional status of young adults, particularly young women, are of particular concern [Scientific Advisory Committee on Nutrition, 2008c] (see Appendix 2 for details) and findings from the Southampton Women's Survey (SWS) indicate that there is little change in diet in the period before conception into early pregnancy [Crozier et al., 2009]. These findings suggest that many young women could be constrained in their ability to meet the nutritional demands of pregnancy

6.4.1.1   Overall dietary quality

406.   Dietary quality potentially influences effects on the offspring as much as quantity. Key findings from national dietary surveys previously highlighted by SACN are outlined in Appendix 2. These data show that a high proportion of women consume high levels of saturated fat and sugar, while non-starch polysaccharide (NSP) and fish consumption are well below the recommended levels.

407.   In a study of non-pregnant women aged 20-34 years living in Southampton (the Southampton Women's Survey), a "prudent" score for dietary pattern was devised to assess accordance with guidelines for healthy eating. Women with high scores, representing greater concordance with current guidelines, were characterised as consuming more fruits, vegetables and wholemeal bread. Those with low scores consumed more white bread and chips, added sugar and full-fat dairy products. The study found that women with lower educational attainment had lower prudent scores. This was the most influential factor, but it was not simply a result of lower income [Robinson *et al.*, 2004]. Results from the Low Income Diet and Nutrition Survey (LIDNS) (see Appendix 2), in which the types and quantities of many foods eaten and patterns of nutrient intake were very similar to the general population, support this finding.

408.   National data show that high proportions of young women also have low intakes and biochemical status for several micronutrients [Scientific Advisory Committee on Nutrition, 2008c] (see Appendix 2 for details). Several small studies have also reported low micronutrient intakes in pregnant women in the UK, particularly those from more socially deprived areas [Rees *et al.*, 2005a; Rees *et al.*, 2005b, Mouratidou *et al.*, 2006] (see details in Appendix 2). One study found that the most deprived women consumed diets poorer in protein, fibre, and vitamins and minerals [Haggarty *et al.*, 2009].

409.   Women of lower educational attainment and those from deprived social backgrounds are thus more likely to exhibit poor dietary patterns at conception. Consequently, they are at greater risk of inadequate status for some micronutrients, particularly those considered later in section 6.4.1.3.

410.   An adequate intake of vitamins and minerals is particularly important for adolescent girls in preparation for motherhood and during the childbearing years of all women (particularly while they are pregnant and lactating) to ensure micronutrient status at conception is adequate to support optimum fetal development. During these critical periods, dietary quality can impact greatly on the health of both the mother and the child.

6.4.1.2   Fruit and vegetable consumption

411.   National surveys indicate that a high proportion of young women of childbearing age consume fewer than the recommended five portions of vegetables and fruit each day [Scientific Advisory Committee on Nutrition, 2008c; Aresu *et al.*, 2010] (see Appendix 2 for details). The 2009 Health Survey for England trends data showed that reported fruit and vegetable consumption (mean number of

portions) in women aged 16-44 remained similar or fell in 2009 compared to the previous years[xxxvi] [Aresu *et al.*, 2010].

412.   Fruit and vegetables are particularly rich in vitamin C. Although vitamin C intakes and status were adequate in women of all ages in NDNS, relatively high proportions of women in LIDNS (i.e. from low-income groups) had low biochemical status for vitamin C[xxxvii] although intakes were adequate. In addition, a comparison of data from LIDNS and NDNS suggests that the low-income population consume fewer portions of fruit and vegetables than the general population (Appendix 2).

413.   National surveys have shown that vitamin A intakes in a substantial number of women of childbearing age are below the LRNI, which suggests some women may be at risk of deficiency at the start of pregnancy, although there was no evidence of low vitamin A status based on plasma retinol levels. Pregnant women are advised to avoid taking supplements containing preformed vitamin A (retinol) and to also avoid consuming liver or liver products. This advice is based on the risk of teratogenesis associated with retinol consumption at doses exceeding 3000µg retinol equivalents (RE) per day [Expert Group on Vitamins and Minerals, 2003]. Fruits and vegetables are a good source of β-carotene (provitamin A), which is converted to retinol in the body and does not pose a risk of teratogenesis.

6.4.1.3 Specific nutrients causing concern

6.4.1.3.1 Folic acid

414.   The association between maternal folate status and the development of fetal neural tube defects (NTD) is well established [Scientific Advisory Committee on Nutrition, 2006]. Since the amount of folic acid required to minimise the risk of developing NTDs cannot be achieved through dietary measures alone, folic acid supplementation is recommended and proven to be highly effective in optimising folate status.

415.   All women who could become pregnant are advised to take a 400µg/d folic acid supplement prior to conception and until the twelfth week of pregnancy to reduce the risk of neural tube defects, such as spina bifida, in unborn babies [Scientific Advisory Committee on Nutrition, 2006]. Certain groups at increased risk, such as those with a past history of NTD affected pregnancies, are advised to take 5mg daily.

416.   There is some evidence of marginal folate status in young women [Scientific Advisory Committee on Nutrition, 2008c]. Several reports from British studies of pregnant women have also indicated that total folate intake is lower than the RNI of 300µg/d in pregnant women [Haste *et al.*, 1991; Wynn *et al.*, 1991; Anderson *et al.*, 1995; Robinson *et al.*, 1996; Mathews & Neil, 1998; Rogers *et al.*, 1998].

417.   Despite promotion of folic acid supplementation, a high proportion of women appear to be unaware of the recommendation and do not take supplements

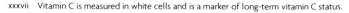

xxxvi   In women aged 16-24, mean number of portions fell from 3.2 in 2007 to 3.1 in 2008 and 3.1 in 2009, 4.0 to 3.7 to 3.6 in women aged 25-34, and 4.0 to 3.8 to 3.7 in women aged 35-44.

xxxvii   Vitamin C is measured in white cells and is a marker of long-term vitamin C status.

(evidence from national surveys including the Infant Feeding Survey, Health Survey for England and also the Southampton Women's Survey Study Group; see Appendix 2 for details). Furthermore, about half of pregnancies are unplanned, the proportion in adolescents being particularly high. These young women are at greater risk of folate deficiency and hence NTD affected pregnancy. SACN has recommended mandatory fortification of flour with folic acid in the UK as an effective measure to prevent pregnancies affected by NTDs [Scientific Advisory Committee on Nutrition, 2009]. This measure is currently under consideration.

418. It is possible that low folate status during pregnancy has more widespread implications. Some epidemiological evidence suggests that a mother with low folate status may also be at risk of preterm delivery, having low birthweight babies or babies born small for gestational age (see Chapter 3.1.4.1.2). Moreover, there is evidence from feeding studies in animals that alteration of methylation status through varying dietary intake of folate may exacerbate or attenuate the effects of dietary protein restriction (see Chapter 5.2). High folate intakes in vitamin B_{12} deficient mothers have been associated with an increased risk of insulin resistance in the offspring [Yajnik et al., 2008] (results from the Pune Maternal Nutrition Study - see section 3.1.4.1.5). These findings indicate that interaction may occur between vitamins involved in the methylation cycle and emphasise the importance of achieving a better understanding of dietary balance in pregnancy.

6.4.1.3.2 Vitamin D

419. As outlined previously by SACN [Scientific Advisory Committee on Nutrition, 2007b], poor maternal vitamin D status adversely affects fetal and Infant growth and development. In particular, It Is associated with poor bone development and rickets in the offspring (Chapter 4.6.1). The vitamin D RNI for pregnant and lactating women is 10µg/d [Department of Health, 1991]. Both SACN and NICE have emphasised the need for all pregnant and lactating women to take a daily supplement of vitamin D, both to ensure their own requirement for vitamin D is met and to build fetal stores for early infancy [Scientific Advisory Committee on Nutrition, 2007b; National Institute for Health and Clinical Excellence, 2008a; National Institute for Health and Clinical Excellence, 2008b].

420. National surveys show that a high proportion of women are likely to begin pregnancy with low vitamin D status. In particular, women of South Asian origin and younger women appear to be at most risk [Scientific Advisory Committee on Nutrition, 2007b; Scientific Advisory Committee on Nutrition, 2008c] (see Appendix 2 for details). British studies have consistently reported average vitamin D intakes to be lower than the RNI during pregnancy [Wynn et al., 1991; Anderson et al., 1995; Robinson et al., 1996; Mathews & Neil, 1998], and low biochemical vitamin D status is widespread [Javaid et al., 2006; Datta et al., 2002; Shenoy et al., 2005]. Whilst it is well recognised that ethnic minority groups are particularly vulnerable to vitamin D deficiency [Scientific Advisory Committee on Nutrition, 2007b], a high proportion of women of White European ancestry also have low biochemical status, particularly at Northerly latitudes in the UK.

421.	There are no national data on the use of vitamin D supplements during pregnancy, but some evidence suggests that usage is low [Javaid et al., 2006] and there appears to be lack of awareness of the current recommendations [Scientific Advisory Committee on Nutrition, 2007b] (also see Appendix 2 for details).

6.4.1.3.3 Iron

422.	There is no national information on iron intakes of pregnant women in the UK, but intakes in non-pregnant women of childbearing age are frequently below recommended levels [Scientific Advisory Committee on Nutrition, 2008c] (see Appendix 2). Several reports from small British studies of pregnant women have indicated that mean iron intakes were below the RNI [Haste et al., 1991; Wynn et al., 1991; Anderson et al., 1995; Robinson et al., 1996; Rogers et al., 1998]. However, there is little correlation between iron intake and iron status measured by haemoglobin [Department of Health, 2002].

423.	There is a lack of national data on the prevalence of iron deficiency in pregnancy, but local studies in the United Kingdom suggest the prevalence of low haemoglobin concentration in early gestation is low [Murphy et al., 1986; Godfrey et al., 1991; Robinson et al., 1998]. The co-existence of apparently low iron intakes with infrequency of anaemia suggests the current DRVs for iron may be inappropriately high. They may not account adequately for adaptation to meet requirements through increased intestinal absorption [Scientific Advisory Committee on Nutrition, 2010]. The strong inverse correlation between parity and ferritin levels may nevertheless indicate that multiparous mothers have reduced iron stores [Robinson et al., 1998].

424.	In 2008, NICE recommended that iron supplementation should not be offered routinely to pregnant women but should be considered for women identified with haemoglobin levels below 110g/L in the first trimester and 105g/L at 28 weeks of gestation. This recommendation has been supported by SACN [Scientific Advisory Committee on Nutrition, 2010]. Despite these recommendations there is evidence that a high proportion of women currently consume iron supplements during pregnancy (see Appendix 2).

6.5   BMI trends, obesity and pregnancy outcome

425.	Section 3.1.4.2 reviewed the adverse effects of maternal obesity and overweight on perinatal risk and later health of the offspring.

6.5.1   Prevalence of overweight and obesity in the UK

426.	There has been an overall increase in overweight and obesity in both adults and children in the UK [Government Office for Science, 2007]. In 2009, 16% of boys and 15% of girls aged 2-15 years were classed as obese[xxxviii], an overall increase from 11% of boys and 12% of girls in 1995 [Aresu et al., 2010] (Figure 16). However, there are indications that the trend has slowed over the last two to three years.

---

xxxviii   The UK National BMI percentiles are used to define overweight and obesity in children as at or over the 85th or 95th BMI percentiles respectively of the 1990 reference population.

Figure 16 – Overweight and obesity prevalence of children aged 2-15 (1995-2009) by sex (three year moving averages)

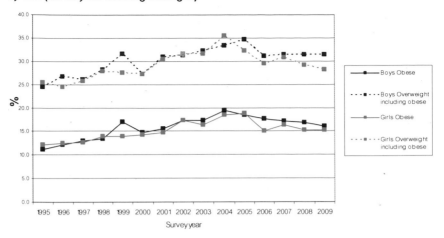

From Health Survey for England 2009 [Aresu et al., 2010]

427. In 2009, 56.7% of women were either overweight or obese[xxxix] [Aresu et al., 2010]. The proportion of women who are obese (BMI 30 or over) has increased from 16.4% in 1993 to 23.9% in 2009, although this had dropped from 24.9% in 2008 (Figure 17). The NDNS and LIDNS also identified a high proportion of females aged 11-49 years as overweight or obese (Appendix 2, Tables 15 and 16)[xl].

Figure 17 – Percentage women overweight or obese (defined by BMI) by survey year and age of woman

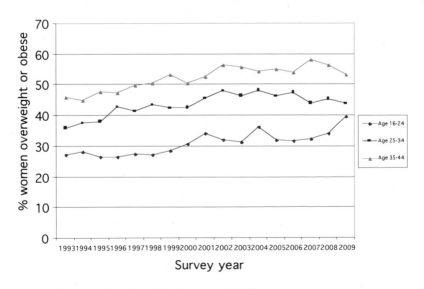

From Health Survey for England 2009 [Aresu et al., 2010]

xxxix   36.9% of women aged 16-24 were obese, 43.7% of women aged 25-34, and 53.3% of women aged 35-44.

xl   In women, overweight and obese are classified as a BMI of 25 and 30, respectively. In adolescents, overweight and obese are classified as BMI >85th <95th BMI centile and BMI >95th BMI centile, respectively.

428. Foresight has estimated that the prevalence of obesity in children will reach 25% by 2050, with a further 40% overweight [Government Office for Science, 2007]. It has been predicted that 60% per cent of men and 50% of women will be obese by 2050 and a further 35% will be overweight.

429. There are no national statistics about the prevalence of obesity in pregnancy in the UK, but according to statistics from the 2006 Health Survey for England, 18% of women in England were obese at the start of pregnancy [National Institute for Health and Clinical Excellence, 2010].

430. Some local studies have also been published. A retrospective study of 287,213 pregnant women in London found that 28% and 11% were overweight or obese respectively [Sebire et al., 2001]. Similarly, 19% of 30,167 pregnant women in Manchester were obese [Shah et al., 2005].

431. Another study observing trends among 36,821 pregnant women in Middlesborough found that the incidence of maternal obesity at the start of pregnancy had increased significantly from 9.9% to 16.0% between 1990 and 2004 (p<0.01). The study also observed significant relationships between maternal obesity, deprivation, increasing age and parity. It was predicted that 22% of pregnant women will be obese by 2010 [Heslehurst et al., 2007].

432. Findings from the United Kingdom Obstetric Surveillance System for rare events in pregnancy (UKOSS) show that 1 in every 1000 pregnant women in the UK has a BMI >50 kg/m^2 or weight >140kg. Nationally around 600 pregnancies are affected each year [National Perinatal Epidemiology Unit, 2007].

6.5.2   Implications for pregnancy and future generations

433. The increasing prevalence of childhood obesity is expected to impact on the risk of adult morbidity [Owen et al., 2009b]. Obesity in childhood increases subsequent risk of obesity and associated diseases in adults (Chapter 4.3.2), and it is well known that obesity is associated with an increased risk of premature death [Government Office for Science, 2007; National Institute for Health and Clinical Excellence, 2010]. Those who gain weight most rapidly, are heaviest during infancy, or are at the highest end of the BMI distribution appear to be at increased risk of type 2 diabetes and impaired glucose intolerance in adult life (section 4.4.2). They may also be at increased risk of CHD in adulthood (section 4.2.1.2). Some evidence identifies those who are thinnest in infancy and undergo a rapid increase in BMI in early childhood as being at greatest risk.

434. Both obese women and their babies are at increased risk of pregnancy-related complications [Stephansson et al., 2001; Myles et al., 2002; Cedegran & Kallen, 2003; Watkins et al., 2003; Lashen et al., 2004; Weiss et al., 2004; Kristensen et al., 2005; Ray et al., 2005; Shah et al., 2005; Usha et al., 2005]. Risks for the mother include maternal death or severe morbidity, pre-eclampsia, gestational diabetes and thromboembolism, and for the baby, stillbirth, neonatal death, congenital abnormalities, and preterm birth [Lewis, 2007].

435. Maternal obesity increases the adiposity of the fetus and the newborn baby. This is exacerbated further if maternal obesity is complicated by gestational diabetes, where glucose freely crosses the placenta, stimulates insulin secretion and adipose tissue deposition (section 3.1.4.2). The long-term implications for the offspring are not clear.

436. NICE has issued public health guidance on dietary and physical activity interventions for weight management in pregnancy and after childbirth. They highlight the importance of achieving a healthy weight before pregnancy and the health risks of being overweight or obese during pregnancy [National Institute of Health and Clinical Excellence, 2010]. Clearly, efforts to attain this goal must begin in early life. They also advise that the additional energy requirements for breastfeeding may help some women return to their pre-pregnancy weight.

437. The Institute of Medicine (IOM) recommends that healthy women in the US who are within the normal BMI range (BMI 18.5-24.9) should gain 11.5kg during pregnancy, those overweight (BMI 25-29.9) should gain 7-11.5kg and obese women (BMI >30) should gain only 5-9kg [Rasmussen & Yaktine, 2009]. However, NICE has stated that these recommendations are based on observational data and are not validated by interventions, and so did not therefore endorse these. Furthermore, they are developed for the US population and it is not clear if these would be applicable to other populations [National Institute of Health and Clinical Excellence, 2010].

6.6   Summary

438 Many adults and children in the UK have diets of poor quality. In the context of reproduction, the impact of energy dense, nutrient poor diets on women and children is of particular concern. In general, the evidence indicates co-existence of excessive consumption of energy from refined carbohydrate and saturated fat, with insufficient intake of vegetables, fruit, and oily fish. In consequence, there is a rising prevalence of obesity, coupled with concern about micronutrient status.

439. In the NDNS, women aged 19-24 years were identified as being at particular risk of poor dietary variety and low nutrient intake and biochemical status [Scientific Advisory Committee on Nutrition, 2008c]. The LIDNS indicated similar concerns although some were more marked in the lower income population, for example fruit and vegetable consumption, fibre consumption and intake of some minerals. Low uptake of folic acid supplements amongst women who could become pregnant, and apparent low uptake of vitamin D during pregnancy and lactation are both issues of increasing concern.

440. Maternal obesity represents an important and modifiable risk factor for adverse pregnancy outcome.

441. A mother's educational attainment and income remain important predictors of her own dietary choices and infant feeding behaviour. Past public health interventions focussed on the provision of food supplements during pregnancy or provision of infant formula after birth.

442. There is a lack of information about reasons for ethnic variation in birthweight in the UK, particularly persistence of a greater incidence of low birthweight among women of South Asian origin.

443. There is also a lack of national data to describe the dietary intake and nutritional status of pregnant and breastfeeding women, and of children aged less than 18 months.

7 Overall Summary and Conclusions

444. The evidence associating early life nutrition with later risk of chronic disease comes from many sources and is variable in quality. However, both observational studies in humans and experimental studies in both animals and humans give cause for concern about the later health consequences of compromised or excessive nutrient supply during early growth and development.

445. Most of the human evidence is observational; such studies demonstrate associations, which may or may not be causal, because associations are susceptible to confounding by genetic, environmental and behavioural factors at different stages of the life course (Chapter 4). Importantly, risk of chronic disease is also influenced by factors other than those in early life, including genetic predisposition to disease and a number of modifiable risk factors in adolescence and adulthood.

446. Experimental interventions help to affirm observational findings (Chapter 5). However, the length of the human lifespan poses major methodological challenges to the conduct of intervention studies, but markers of later risk may be used as outcomes. Intervention studies in this context are also contraindicated on the grounds of ethical considerations. Animal models also provide insight.

447. Epidemiological studies involve prospective or retrospective collection of data. These are complementary approaches with different strengths and weaknesses (Chapter 2). In retrospective studies, disease outcomes are known but measures of early life exposures may be weak. Generalisation to contemporary circumstances can also be questionable. Prospective studies more accurately characterise early nutrient exposure and growth but, as with human intervention studies, it may be necessary to infer risk by measuring intermediate markers of later health outcomes. Furthermore, studies from developing countries are not always applicable in the UK context.

Early growth and development (Chapter 3)

448. Growth is a regulated process by which the organism increases in mass, size and complexity. During growth, there are substantial changes in the distribution, architecture and relative amounts of body tissues. These are manifested as developmental changes in metabolic capacity. The maintenance of adequate pre- and postnatal nutrient supply during growth is essential to support these processes.

449. Experimental studies in animals have demonstrated the existence of "critical periods" in early development during which alteration of nutrient supply may alter structure and function irreversibly. This phenomenon has been labelled "nutritional programming". It offers opportunities for intervention, which may reduce the risk of chronic disease in later life.

450. Characterisation of underlying processes requires a developmental perspective that integrates nutrient requirements and supply, composition and distribution of tissues within the body, and functional or metabolic capacity at the whole body and cellular level.

451. The exact relationship between birthweight and chronic disease risk is complex. Observational studies have shown relationships between birthweight and risk of chronic diseases in adult life. The observed relationships vary in strength and consistency; these are not confined to the extremes, and risk tends to be graded across the normal birthweight range. The shape of the association is not clear and the evidence does not allow clear definition of thresholds for healthy birthweight. Associations that have been shown tend to be of modest public health impact. However, extremes of birthweight may carry their own risk.

452. Current risk factors explain a much greater proportion of the variance in chronic disease risk than birthweight. This may be partly explained by the observation that birthweight alone is a weak measure of fetal nutrient supply and *in utero* experience.

453. Although a widely collected and useful measure of pregnancy outcome, birthweight is influenced by many variables other than fetal nutrient supply. These include maternal height, weight, parity, ethnicity and exposure to environmental factors such as alcohol and tobacco smoke. Fetuses may achieve comparable birthweight through different gestational growth trajectories.

454. Infants of comparable birthweight vary in their body composition and metabolic capacity. Animal models of nutrient restriction during pregnancy have confirmed that body composition and metabolic capacity may be altered independently of birthweight. Better understanding of body composition in the human newborn is required to explain relationships between birthweight and risk of chronic disease in adult life.

455. During normal pregnancy, maternal adaptations ensure that fetal nutrient supply is preserved when maternal dietary intake varies. These adaptations may not compensate adequately under extreme conditions such as famine. Both experimental interventions in animals and human epidemiological data from famine conditions, suggest that the timing of maternal nutrient and energy restriction in pregnancy affects fetal outcome. The changes observed can be plausibly related to the timing of organ development.

456. When fetal growth is restricted there is a tendency for early postnatal growth to be accelerated. This is known as "catch-up" or "compensatory" growth. During this process, the normal proportionate distribution and relative weight of tissues and organ systems may be disrupted. Consequent alterations in body composition may be mirrored in altered metabolic function and chronic disease risk. The tendency for "catch-up" to occur makes independent effects of pre- and postnatal nutrient supply on chronic disease risk hard to separate.

Impact of early nutrition on adult health: epidemiological studies (Chapter 4)

457.	The majority of studies show modest inverse associations between birthweight, and the incidence of adult cardiovascular disease (CVD) or indicators of increased CVD risk (blood pressure, serum cholesterol) (section 4.2). Lower birthweight, lower weight at one year, and higher body mass index (BMI) in childhood together are associated with a greater risk of CVD.

458.	Higher birthweight is associated with higher BMI in later life though there remains some doubt about what BMI reflects in this context. The few studies of body composition that have been able to resolve separately the fat and lean mass components, suggest that high birthweight may later be associated with relatively greater lean mass, whereas low birthweight is associated with relatively greater fat mass (section 4.3).

459.	Overall, lower birthweight is also associated with increased risk of subsequent type 2 diabetes, though there may also be increased risk at the upper end of the birthweight distribution too (section 4.4.1).

460.	Impaired glucose tolerance or diabetes is associated with low BMI up to the age of 2 years, followed by an early "adiposity rebound" and accelerated increase in BMI through childhood (section 4.4.2).

461.	Adults who were not breastfed as infants have slightly higher blood pressure and serum total cholesterol concentrations (sections 4.2.2.3 and 4.2.3.2). They are also at greater risk of type 2 diabetes (section 4.4.3) and more likely to be obese (i.e. show increased BMI in later life) (section 4.3.3). The observational evidence that infant feeding influences subsequent cardiovascular mortality is inconsistent (section 4.2.1.3). This may reflect inadequate recall of the duration and exclusivity of breastfeeding, and infant feeding practices generally.

462.	Greater birthweight is associated with an increase in risk of certain cancers in later life, notably breast cancer (particularly in premenopausal women) (section 4.5.2.1) and child leukaemia (section 4.5.1.2). There is also consistent evidence that taller height during childhood and adolescence, and more rapid height gain, are associated with an increased risk of premenopausal breast cancer (section 4.5.2.2). Conversely, greater body fatness during childhood and adolescence is associated with a reduced risk of breast cancer (particularly premenopausal breast cancer) (section 4.5.2.2).

463.	A low rate of childhood growth (i.e. height and weight) may also be a risk factor for later hip fracture (section 4.6.3). There is also some evidence that increased maternal UVB exposure and circulating 25(OH) vitamin D concentrations are positively associated with offspring bone size in later childhood, but the relationship with maternal calcium intake or the effects of maternal calcium supplementation on offspring bone size are not clear (section 4.6.1).

464. The review of the epidemiology considered specific chronic disease outcomes as an illustrative process. Further consideration of excluded outcomes would unlikely allow any more definitive conclusions to be drawn. Although observational data suggest associations between certain early life exposures and chronic disease outcomes in adulthood, and there is some evidence to explain underlying mechanisms, it is difficult to detect and quantify meaningful effect sizes for these associations.

Putative mechanisms and animal models (Chapter 5)

465. RCTs in preterm infants (of very low birthweight) showed slower growth in length and weight in the early years when fed human donor milk compared to those fed a nutrient dense infant formula. However, subsequent weight, length and other physical parameters were similar at 7-8 years of age.

466. A few studies have randomly allocated non-breastfed infants to alternative diets (section 5.1). For example, term infants randomly allocated to receive a low sodium diet during the first six months of life showed a lower systolic blood pressure during infancy and adolescence. Preterm infants randomly allocated to receive human donor milk, as opposed to preterm formula, had lower mean and diastolic blood pressure in adolescence. Such studies confirm that early feeding practices and nutrient intake can exert long-term effects on cardiovascular risk.

467. These findings are consistent with the hypothesis that nutrient exposure during late gestation or early life can alter the susceptibility of human infants to chronic disease in adult life.

468. Experimental studies of nutrient restriction during pregnancy and early life have principally been conducted in animal models (section 5.2). Restriction of macronutrient or micronutrient supply, particularly during late gestation, can reduce birthweight and predispose offspring to hypertension and glucose intolerance. It is important to recognise that varying intake within the range normally encountered by pregnant animals is sufficient to affect these changes.

469. Differing patterns of nutrient restriction in animals may lead to similar phenotypic changes. This suggests that it is dietary imbalance which leads to disruption in fetal development and consequential irreversible alteration of phenotype, not deficiency of a specific nutrient.

470. In rats, restriction of protein intake during pregnancy causes endothelial dysfunction and hypertension in the offspring. It also modifies offspring metabolic pathways including those involved in glucocorticoid and lipid metabolism. Concurrent supplementation with glycine or folic acid abolishes these effects.

471. Dietary manipulation of methylation status in pregnant mice has induced changes in several observable characteristics, for example coat colour. It is postulated that the effects of folic acid or glycine supplementation on offspring phenotype in other species are attributable to alteration of methylation cycle activity.

472. Dietary protein restriction in pregnant rats reduced expression of the hepatic glucorticoid receptor (GR) and peroxisome peripheral activated receptor α (PPARα) in the offspring. A five-fold increase in the folic acid content of the diet increased expression and an associated increase in methylation of the GR and PPARα promoters was noted.

473. Dietary intervention in pregnant animals can therefore induce permanent structural and functional changes in the offspring through epigenetic modification of the genome.

474. The role of epigenetics in human disease is becoming more widely appreciated. Altered methylation of DNA has been associated with some cancers and atherosclerosis.

475. In humans, the dose-response relationships that might result in phenotypic changes similar to those demonstrated in animals are still unclear.

Implications of nutritional status of UK adults for reproduction (Chapter 6)

476. National survey data have consistently indicated that many adults and children in the UK, particularly those socially or educationally deprived, have diets of poor quality. In the context of reproduction, the impact of energy dense diets of low micronutrient content on women and girls is of particular concern. Ongoing national surveys[xli] will provide further insight into the diet and nutritional status of the UK population.

477. The rising prevalence of obesity in girls and young women represents an important and modifiable risk factor for adverse pregnancy outcome.

478. Controlled studies in human pregnancy have not been conducted to allow identification of maternal dietary interventions that effectively reduce risk of adult chronic disease in the offspring.

---

xli   Including the government funded National Diet and Nutrition Survey (NDNS) Rolling Programme, and the Diet and Nutrition Survey of Infants and Young Children (DNSIYC) (due to report in 2012).

8 Recommendations

8.1 Public health recommendations

R1. Optimisation of fetal development requires the achievement of adequate nutritional status of the mother prior to conception. Interventions to reduce chronic disease risk in future generations should address dietary and lifestyle change in infancy and adolescence, to ensure adequate nutrition throughout adolescent and reproductive years and in order to improve women's reproductive health.

R2. Efforts to improve diet quality will need to address health inequalities and consider the diet as a whole without neglecting the importance of supplementation with folic acid and vitamin D. Existing advice to increase fruit and vegetable consumption is designed to improve the overall micronutrient status of women along with appropriate folic acid and vitamin D supplementation.

R3. It is particularly important that adolescent and young adult women achieve a body composition and metabolic capacity capable of meeting the stresses of pregnancy as well as their own requirements. This will help to address the health and economic implications of the rising prevalence of maternal obesity for future generations.

R4. There is a need to increase appreciation of the reproductive risks associated with excess maternal body weight and to support women in achieving and maintaining a healthy weight in preparation for pregnancy.

R5. The increased nutritional vulnerability of underweight women needs to be addressed. There is also a need to recognise the increased nutrient demands on adolescent and young women who become pregnant before completing their own growth.

R6. Strategies that promote, protect and support exclusive breastfeeding for around the first six months of an infant's life should be enhanced, and should recognise the benefits for long-term health. The greatest impact is likely to be achieved by intervening in the early postnatal weeks, when the rate of discontinuation is greatest.

8.2 Research recommendations

R7. Large, longitudinal cohort studies capable of characterising relationships between early life nutritional exposures and adult chronic disease risk should incorporate measures of pre-conceptional nutritional status, fetal and placental growth, offspring body composition and metabolic competence. Such data will better characterise patterns of pre- and post-natal growth associated with greatest risk of adult chronic disease.

R8.   Consideration should be given to building a longitudinal element into national surveys of diet and nutrition in the UK. Repeated measures of body weight and size and dietary intake could be incorporated and linked to health outcome data. The National Diet and Nutrition Survey programme should also consider recruitment of pregnant and breastfeeding women.

R9.   Clinical trials investigating changes to the composition of infant formula should incorporate follow-up to capture long-term outcomes.

R10.   The causes and consequences of variation in birthweight between ethnic groups need to be better understood, particularly their implications for body composition and metabolic competence. There is an associated need to measure trends in these outcomes as succeeding generations are born in the UK.

R11.   Further human research, particularly from intervention studies, is required to understand how maternal body weight and weight gain during pregnancy are related to maternal and offspring health outcome.

R12.   Experimental studies in animal models are required to expand understanding of the mechanisms that explain observed associations between nutrition in early life and subsequent chronic disease outcomes. Such studies would help to identify predictive markers of altered function at molecular, cellular, tissue and whole-body level. These phenotypic markers may have application to human studies.

9 Glossary

"Adiposity rebound"   The point at which BMI begins to increase with age following the nadir observed in the middle childhood years. On average this is observed at about 6 years of age but occurs earlier in relatively heavy children and later in those who are relatively light.

Birth length   The length of a newborn baby from head to heels when the legs are fully extended (*syn.* "crown-heel length").

Birthweight   The weight of an infant at birth.

Body mass index (BMI)   An individual's weight in kilograms divided by the square of height in metres (kg/m^2). Often used as an indicator of adiposity, with recognised limitations [Pietrobelli *et al.*, 1998].

Bottle-feeding   Feeding an infant from a bottle, whatever is in the bottle, including expressed breastmilk, water, formula, etc.

Canalisation   As applied to the study of growth the term describes the tendency to follow a genetically-determined trajectory given optimal health conditions and nutrient supply.

Cardiovascular disease (CVD)   Cardiovascular disease is the most common cause of death in the UK and includes coronary heart disease (CHD), angina, heart attack and stroke.

Catch-up growth (or compensatory growth)   Rapid growth following a period of restriction. Ultimately, it may redress wholly or partly the accrued deficit in weight or size though there may be consequences for body composition and metabolic capacity.

Cohort study   Systematic follow-up of a group of people for a defined period of time or until a specified event. Also known as a longitudinal study. A cohort study may collect data prospectively or retrospectively.

Complementary feeding   The process by which mothers give foods additional to breastmilk or infant formula.

DXA (dual energy x-ray absorptiometry).   A technique used to measure the mineral content of bones or the distribution and relative amounts of soft tissues. DXA exposes the body or parts of the body to very low doses of ionising radiation in the form of dual beams which differ in energy value.

DNA-methylation	DNA methylation involves the addition of a methyl group to DNA - for example, to the number 5 carbon of the cytosine pyrimidine ring, which has a specific effect of reducing gene expression.
Diabetes	A metabolic disorder involving impaired metabolism of glucose due to either failure of secretion of the hormone insulin, *insulin-dependent or type 1 diabetes*, OR impaired responses of tissues to insulin, *non-insulin-dependent or type 2 diabetes*. See also **gestational diabetes**.
Embryogenesis	The process by which the embryo is formed and developed.
Epigenetics	Cellular mechanisms that confer stability of gene expression during development. Epigenetic marking imprints gene expression in somatic tissues and these marks subsequently take form as differential DNA methylation.
Exclusive breastfeeding	The infant receives only breastmilk and may be given drops or syrups consisting of vitamins, mineral supplements or medicines but no other food or liquids. UK Health Departments recommend exclusive breastfeeding for the first six months of an infant's life [Department of Health, 2003].
Formula, Infant formula	A breastmilk substitute commercially manufactured to Codex Alimentarius or European Union standards.
Genetic polymorphism	Variability in one or more base pairs in the DNA gene sequence encoding a specific protein. This results in the substitution of different amino acids in that protein, which may subtly alter its function. The most common type of polymorphism involves variation at a single base pair. This is called a single nucleotide polymorphism, or SNP.
Genomic imprinting	*Genomic imprinting* refers to the epigenetic marking of the parental origin of certain chromosomal domains and takes place at a small subset of genes termed imprinted genes.
Genotype	The genetic constitution of an individual, as distinct from its expressed features or *phenotype*.
Gestational age	The age of a fetus calculated from the first day of the mother's last menstrual period.
Gestational diabetes	Gestational diabetes mellitus (GDM) is defined as any degree of glucose intolerance with onset or first recognition during pregnancy.

Hazard ratio (HR)	The ratio of *hazard rates* at a single time between two groups. Hazard ratios can provide a good way to present the relative effects of two treatments on the health outcome of interest. **Hazard Rate** is the probability (per time unit) that a subject (without the health outcome of interest at the beginning of the time interval) will have the health outcome of interest in that time interval.
Head circumference	The circumference of the head measured at the level of the frontal and occipital prominences, its largest diameter.
Histone	A protein rich in arginine and lysine that occurs mainly in the cell nucleus and is concerned with the regulation of DNA expression.
Infant	A child not more than one year of age.
Intervention Study	Comparison of an outcome (e.g. disease) between two or more groups deliberately subjected to different exposures (e.g. dietary modification or nutrient supplementation).
Intrauterine Growth Restriction (IUGR)	The faltering of growth *in utero*.
Longitudinal Study	In a longitudinal study, individual subjects are followed through time with continuous or repeated monitoring exposures, health outcomes, or both.
Low birthweight (LBW)	Birthweight less than 2.5kg. Infants may be low birthweight because they are born too early or are unduly small for gestational age.
Lower reference nutrient intake (LRNI)	The estimated average daily intake of a nutrient which can be expected to meet the needs of only 2.5% of a healthy population. Values set may vary according to age, gender and physiological state (e.g. pregnancy or breastfeeding).
Macronutrients	Nutrients that provide energy, including fat, protein and carbohydrate.
Metabolic competence	The capability of an individual, organ or system to carry out some metabolic function. The term "metabolic capacity" describes the individual's maximal capability.

Metabolic syndrome	The metabolic syndrome describes the clustering of factors including dyslipidaemia, glucose intolerance and hypertension with central adiposity. Diagnosis of metabolic syndrome requires coexistence of three of the following manifestations: waist circumference ≥102 cm (men) or ≥88 cm (women); blood pressure ≥130/85; HDL-cholesterol <40 mg/dL (men) or <50 mg/dL (women); triglycerides ≥150 mg/dL; fasting glucose ≥110 mg/dL.
Meta-analysis	A quantitative pooling of estimates of effect of an exposure on a given outcome, from different studies identified from a systematic review of the literature
Micronutrients	Essential nutrients required by the body in small quantities, including vitamins and minerals.
Mixed feeding	An infant receives both breastmilk and infant formula. *Complementary feeding* (see above) is the process by which mothers give foods additional to breastmilk or infant formula
Nutrient deficiency	Impaired function due to inadequate supply of a nutrient required by the body.
Nutritional status	An individual's position with respect to the maintenance of nutrient homeostasis [Department of Health, 2002]. It is generally assessed by reference to a) energy and nutrient intake and losses, used to estimate the adequacy of dietary supply; b) body composition (e.g. body mass index (BMI), waist-hip ratio and more specific estimates of tissue composition and distribution); and c) metabolic and physiological function (e.g. biochemical and dynamic measures of organ and tissue function) used to assess the metabolic capacity of an individual, organ or system.
Obesity	In adults, defined on the basis of a body mass index (BMI) of >30 kg/m². Children are usually classified as obese by comparing their BMI with a reference population (UK1990 reference) that describes the distribution of BMI within a population by both age and sex. In population surveillance a BMI >95th centile is generally applied; for clinical purposes a BMI >98th centile is more commonly cited.
Odds ratio (OR)	A measure of the risk of an outcome such as cancer, associated with an exposure of interest, used in case-control studies; approximately equivalent to the relative risk [World Cancer Research Fund / American Institute for Cancer Research, 2007].

Overweight	In adults, defined on the basis of a body mass index (BMI) of ›25 kg/m² in adults. Children are usually classified as overweight by comparing their BMI with a reference population (UK1990 reference) that describes the distribution of BMI within a population by both age and sex. For population surveillance a BMI ›85th centile is generally used; for clinical purposes a BMI ›91st centile is more commonly cited.
Phenotype	Observable physical or biochemical characteristics, which represent the distinctive expression of an individual's genotype in a given environment.
Ponderal index (Rohrer)	An index of fatness, often used as a measure of obesity – the body weight in kilograms divided by the height or length in metres cubed (kg/m³).
PPARs	Peroxisome proliferator-activated receptors (PPARs) are a group of nuclear receptor proteins that function as transcription factors regulating the expression of genes. PPARs play essential roles in the regulation of cellular differentiation, development, metabolism (carbohydrate, lipid, protein), and tumorigenesis of higher organisms.
Randomised Controlled Trial (RCT)	A study in which eligible participants are assigned to two or more treatment groups on a random allocation basis. Randomisation assures the play of chance so that all sources of bias, known and unknown, are equally balanced.
Reference nutrient intake (RNI)	The average daily intake of a nutrient sufficient to meet the needs of almost all members (97.5%) of a healthy population. Values set may vary according to age, gender and physiological state (e.g. pregnancy or breastfeeding).
Relative risk (RR)	The ratio of the rate of disease or death among people exposed to a factor, compared to the rate among the unexposed, usually used in cohort studies [World Cancer Research Fund / American Institute for Cancer Research, 2007].
Rickets	Malformation of the skeleton in growing children due to osteomalacia (softening of the bones).
Risk Factor	A factor demonstrated in epidemiological studies to influence the likelihood of disease in groups of the population.

Skinfold thickness	An indicator of the amount of subcutaneous fat deposited. Skinfold thickness is commonly measured at four sites: biceps (midpoint of front upper arm), triceps (midpoint of back upper arm), sub-scapular (directly below point of shoulder blade at an angle of 45 degrees), and supra-iliac (directly above iliac crest in mid-axillary line). Measurements can be summed and used, or used to calculate % body fat.
Small for gestational age (SGA)	A newborn whose weight falls below a given threshold (most commonly <10th percentile) on a specified birthweight reference.
Solids	Foods other than breastmilk or formula milk introduced to the infant diet at the commencement of complementary feeding.
Stunting	Impaired growth in height due to chronic under-nutrition.
Systematic Review	An extensive review of published literature on a specific topic using a defined search strategy, with a priori inclusion and exclusion criteria.
Waist to hip ratio	Waist circumference (metres) divided by hip circumference (metres), often used as an indicator of central fat distribution (abdominal fat).
Weaning	The process of expanding the diet to include foods and drinks other than breastmilk or infant formula [Department of Health, 1994]. The term *complementary feeding* is preferred to describe diversification of the diet because "weaning" has also been used to describe curtailment of breastfeeding.
Z-score	The Z-score (or standard deviation (SD) score) is defined as the difference between an observed value for an individual and the median value of the reference population, divided by the standard deviation value of the reference population. Z-scores are used for height, weight and head circumference.

10 References

Abrams B, Altman SL, Pickett KE (2000) Pregnancy weight gain: still controversial. *Am J Clin Nutr* 71: S1233-S1241

Abrams BF, Laros RK (1986) Prepregnancy weight, weight gain, and birth weight. *Am J Obstet Gynecol* 154: 503-509

Ahlgren M, Melbye M, Wohlfahrt J, Sorensen TIA (2004) Growth patterns and the risk of breast cancer in women. *N Engl J Med* 351: 1619-1626

Akre O, Forssell L, Kaijser M, Noren-Nilsson I, Lagergren J, Nyren O, Ekbom A (2006) Perinatal risk factors for cancer of the esophagus and gastric cardia: a nested case-control study. *Cancer Epidemiol Biomarkers Prev* 15: 867-871

Allgrove J (2004) Is nutritional rickets returning? *Arch Dis Child* 89: 699-701

Altman DG, Hytten FE (1989) Intrauterine growth retardation: let's be clear about it. *Br J Obstet Gynaecol* 96: 1127-1132

Anderson A, Campbell D, Shepherd R (1995) The influence of dietary advice on nutrient intake during pregnancy. *Br J Nutr* 15: 105-177

Andersson SW, Bengtsson C, Hallberg L, Lapidus L, Niklasson A, Wallgren A, Hulthen L (2001) Cancer risk in Swedish women: the relation to size at birth. *Br J Cancer* 84: 1193-1198

Arenz S, Ruckerl R, Koletzko B, von Kries R (2004) Breast-feeding and childhood obesity – a systematic review. *Int J Obes Relat Metab Disord* 28: 1247-1256

Aresu M, Bécares L, Brage S, Chaudhury M, Doyle-Francis M, Esliger D, Fuller E, Gunning N, Hall J, Hirani V, Jotangia D, Mindell J, Moody A, Ogunbadejo T, Pickup D, Reilly N, Robinson C, Roth M, Wardle H (2009) *Health Survey for England 2008: Physical activity and fitness*. London: The NHS Information Centre for Health and Social Care

Aresu M, Chaudhury M, Diment E, Fuller E, Gordon-Dseagu V, Gunning N, Mindell J, Nicholson S, Ogunbadejo T, Robinson C, Roderick P, Roth M, Shelton N, Tabassum F, Wardle H (2010) *Health Survey for England 2009: Health and Lifestyles Volume 1*. London: The NHS Information Centre for Health and Social Care

Axelsson IE, Ivarsson SA, Raiha NC (1989) Protein intake in early infancy: effects on plasma amino acid concentrations, insulin metabolism, and growth. *Pediatr Res* 26: 614-617

Baer HJ, Colditz GA, Rosner B, Michels KB, Rich-Edwards JW, Hunter DJ, Willett WC (2005) Body fatness during childhood and adolescence and incidence of breast cancer in premenopausal women: a prospective cohort study. *Breast Cancer Res* 7: R314-R325

Baird J, Fisher D, Lucas P, Kleijnen J, Roberts H, Law C (2005) Being big or growing fast: systematic review of size and growth in infancy and later obesity. *BMJ 331*: 929

Baker PN, Wheeler SJ, Sanders TA, Thomas JE, Hutchinson CJ, Clarke K, Berry JL, Jones RL, Seed PT, Poston L (2009) A prospective study of micronutrient status in adolescent pregnancy. *Am J Cl Nutr* 89(4): 1114-1124

Bakker R, Rifas-Shiman SL, Kleinman KP, Lipshultz SE, Gillman MW (2008) Maternal calcium intake during pregnancy and blood pressure in the offspring at age 3 years: a follow-up analysis of the Project Viva cohort. *Am J Epidemiol* 168(12): 1374-1380

Barker DJ (1998) *Mothers, babies and health in later life*. London: Churchhill Livingstone.

Barker DJ, Bull AR, Osmond C, Simmonds SJ (1990) Fetal and placental size and risk of hypertension in adult life. *BMJ 301*: 259-262

Barker DJ, Eriksson JG, Forsen T, Osmond C (2002) Fetal origins of adult disease: strength of effects and biological basis. *Int J Epidemiol* 31: 1235-1239

Barker DJ, Martyn CN (1992) The maternal and fetal origins of cardiovascular disease. *Journal of Epidemiol Community Health* 46: 8-11

Barker DJ, Martyn CN, Osmond C, Hales CN, Fall CH (1993) Growth *in utero* and serum cholesterol concentrations in adult life. *BMJ 307*: 1524-1527

Barker DJ, Osmond C, Forsen TJ, Kajantie E, Eriksson JG (2005) Trajectories of growth among children who have coronary events as adults. *N Engl J Med* 353: 1802-1809

Barker DJ, Osmond C, Golding J, Kuh D, Wadsworth ME (1989a) Growth *in utero*, blood pressure in childhood and adult life, and mortality from cardiovascular disease. *BMJ* 298: 564-567

Barker DJ, Winter PD, Osmond C, Margetts B, Simmonds SJ (1989b) Weight in infancy and death from ischaemic heart disease. *Lancet* 2: 577-580

Bavdekar A, Yajnik CS, Fall CH, Bapat S, Pandit AN, Deshpande V, Bhave S, Kellingray SD, Joglekar C (1999) Insulin resistance syndrome in 8-year-old Indian children: small at birth, big at 8 years, or both? *Diabetes* 48: 2422-2429

Belizan JM, Villar J, Bergel E, del Pino A, De Fulvio S, Galliano SV, Kattan C (1997) Long term effect of calcium supplementation during pregnancy on the blood pressure of offspring: follow-up of a randomized control trial. *BMJ* 315: 281-285

Bellinger L, Lilley C, Langley-Evans SC (2004) Prenatal exposure to a maternal low-protein diet programmes a preference for high-fat foods in the young adult rat. *Br J Nutr 92*: 513-520

Bennis-Taleb N, Remacle C, Hoet JJ, Reusens B (1999) A low-protein isocaloric diet during gestation affects brain development and alters permanently cerebral cortex blood vessels in rat offspring. *J Nutr* 129: 1613-1619

Benvenisty N, Mencher D, Meyuhas O, Razin A, Reshef L (1985) Sequential changes in DNA methylation patterns of the rat phosphoenolpyruvate carboxykinase gene during development. *Proc Natl Acad Sci USA* 82: 267-271

Benyshek DC, Johnston CS, Martin JF (2006) Glucose metabolism is altered in the adequately-nourished grand-offspring (F3 generation) of rats malnourished during gestation and perinatal life. *Diabetologia* 49: 1117-1119

Berenson GS, Srinivasan SR, Bao W, Newman WP, Tracy RE, Wattigney WA (1998) Association between multiple cardiovascular risk factors and atherosclerosis in children and young adults. The Bogalusa Heart Study. *N Engl J Med* 338: 1650-1656

Berkey CS, Frazier AL, Gardner JD, Colditz GA (1999) Adolescence and breast carcinoma risk. *Cancer* 85: 2400-2409

Bertram CE, Hanson MA (2001) Animal models and programming of the metabolic syndrome. *Br Med Bull* 60: 103-121

Bertram CE, Trowern AR, Copin N, Jackson AA, Whorwood CB (2001) The maternal diet during pregnancy programs altered expression of the glucocorticoid receptor and type 2 11beta-hydroxysteroid dehydrogenase: potential molecular mechanisms underlying the programming of hypertension *in utero*. *Endocrinol* 142: 2841-2853

Bhargava SK, Sachdev HS, Fall CH, Osmond C, Lakshmy R, Barker DJ, Biswas SK, Ramji S, Prabhakaran D, Reddy KS (2004) Relation of serial changes in childhood body-mass index to impaired glucose tolerance in young adulthood. *N Engl J Med* 350: 865-875

Bird A (2002) DNA methylation patterns and epigenetic memory. *Genes Dev* 16: 6-21

Blair EM, Liu Y, de Klerk NH, Lawrence DM (2005) Optimal fetal growth for the Caucasian singleton and assessment of appropriateness of fetal growth: an analysis of a total population perinatal database. *BMC Pediatr* 5: 13

Blake M, Herrick, K, Kelly Y (2003) *Health Survey for England 2002: Maternal and Infant Health*. London: The Stationery Office.

Bloomfield FH, Oliver MH, Harding JE (2006) The late effects of fetal growth patterns. *Arch Dis Child Fetal Neonatal Ed* 91: F299-F304

Boden G (1996) Fuel metabolism in pregnancy and in gestational diabetes mellitus. *Obstet Gynecol Clin North Am* 23: 1-10

Bolling K, Grant C, Hamlyn B, Thornton A (2007) *Infant Feeding Survey 2005*. London: The Information Centre.

Bonsch D, Lenz B, Kornhuber J, Bleich S (2005) DNA hypermethylation of the alpha synuclein promoter in patients with alcoholism. *Neuroreport* 16: 167-170

Bonsch D, Lenz B, Reulbach U, Kornhuber J, Bleich S (2004) Homocysteine associated genomic DNA hypermethylation in patients with chronic alcoholism. *J Neural Transm* 111: 1611-1616

Borch-Johnsen K, Joner G, Mandrup-Poulsen T, Christy M, Zachau-Christiansen B, Kastrup K, Nerup J (1984) Relation between breast-feeding and incidence rates of insulin-dependent diabetes mellitus. *Lancet* 2: 1083-1086

Brameld JM, Buttery PJ, Dawson JM, Harper JM (1998) Nutritional and hormonal control of skeletal-muscle cell growth and differentiation. *Proc Nutr Soc* 57: 207-217

Brawley L, Torrens C, Anthony FW, Itoh S, Wheeler T, Jackson AA, Clough GF, Poston L, Hanson MA (2004) Glycine rectifies vascular dysfunction induced by dietary protein imbalance during pregnancy. *J Physiol* 554: 497-504

Brennan KA, Gopalakrishnan GS, Kurlak L, Rhind SM, Kyle CE, Brooks AN, Rae MT, Olson DM, Stephenson T, Symonds ME (2005) Impact of maternal undernutrition and fetal number on glucocorticoid, growth hormone and insulin-like growth factor receptor mRNA abundance in the ovine fetal kidney. *Reproduction* 129: 151-159

Brion M-J, Leary SD, Lawlor DA, Smith GD, Ness AR (2008a) Modifiable maternal exposures and offspring blood pressure: a review of epidemiological studies of maternal age, diet, and smoking. *Pediatric Research* 63(6): 593-598

Brion M-J, Ness AR, Davey Smith G, Emmett P, Rogers I, Whincup P, Lawlor DA (2008b) Sodium intake in infancy and blood pressure at 7 years: findings from the Avon Longitudinal Study of Parents and Children. *Eur J Clin Nutr* 62: 1162-1169

Brooks AA, Johnson MR, Steer PJ, Pawson ME, Abdalla HI (1995) Birth weight: nature or nurture? *Early Hum Dev* 42: 29-35

Brown JE, Kaye SA, Folsom AR (1992) Parity-related weight change in women *Int J Obes Relat Metab Disord* 16(9): 627-631

Brunner E, Shipley MJ, Blane D, Davey Smith G, Marmot MG (1999) When does cardiovascular risk start? Past and present socioeconomic circumstances and risk factors in adulthood. *J Epidemiol Community Health* 53: 757-764

Burdge GC, Hanson MA, Slater-Jefferies JL, Lillycrop KA (2007a) Epigenetic regulation of transcription: a mechanism for inducing variations in phenotype (fetal programming) by differences in nutrition during early life? *Br J Nutr* 97(6): 1036-1046

Burdge GC, Phillips ES, Dunn RL, Jackson AA, Lillycrop KA (2004) Effect of reduced maternal protein consumption during pregnancy in the rat on plasma lipid concentrations and expression of peroxisomal proliferator-activated receptors in the liver and adipose tissue of the offspring. *Nutr Res* 24: 639-646

Burdge GC, Slater-Jefferies J, Torrens C, Phillips ES, Hanson MA, Lillycrop KA (2007b) Dietary protein restriction of pregnant rats in the F0 generation induces altered methylation of hepatic gene promoters in the adult male offspring in the F1 and F2 generations. *Br J Nutr* 97: 435-439

Byrne CD (2001) Programming other hormones that affect insulin. *British Medical Bulletin* 60: 153-171

Callaghan AL, Moy RJ, Booth IW, Debelle GD, Shaw NJ (2006) Incidence of symptomatic vitamin D deficiency. *Arch Dis Child* 91: 606-607

Cameron N, Preece MA, Cole TJ (2005) Catch up growth or regression to the mean? Recovery from stunting revisited. *Am J Hum Biol* 17: 412-417

Cardwell CR, Patterson CC (2009) Re: "birth weight, early weight gain, and subsequent risk of type 1 diabetes: systematic review and meta-analysis". *Am J Epidemiol* 170(4): 529-530

Castro R, Rivera I, Struys EA, Jansen EE, Ravasco P, Camilo ME, Blom HJ, Jakobs C, Tavares de Almeida I (2003) Increased homocysteine and S-adenosylhomocysteine concentrations and DNA hypomethylation in vascular disease. *Clin Chem* 49: 1292-1296

Catalano PM, Ehrenberg HM (2006) The short- and long-term implications of maternal obesity on the mother and her offspring. *Br J Obstet Gynaecol* 113: 1126-1133

Catalano PM, Huston LP, Thomas AJ, Fung CM (1998) Effect of maternal metabolism on fetal growth and body composition. *Diabetes Care* 21: B85-B90

Cedegran MI, Kallen BA (2003) Maternal obesity and infant heart defects. *Obes Res* 11: 1065-1071

Ceesay SM, Prentice AM, Cole TJ, Foord F, Poskitt EME, Weaver LT, Whitehead RG (1997) Effects on birth weight and perinatal mortality of maternal dietary supplements in rural Gambia: 5 year randomised controlled trial. *BMJ* 315: 786-790

Charles DH, Ness AR, Campbell D, Smith GD, Whitley E, Hall MH (2005) Folic acid supplements in pregnancy and birth outcome: re-analysis of a large randomised controlled trial and update of Cochrane review. *Paediatr Perinat Epidemiol* 19: 112-124

Chaudhury M, Falaschetti E, Fuller E, Mackenzie H, Mindell J, Nicholson S, Pickup D, Roth M, Scholes S, Tabassum F, Thompson J, Wardle H (2008) *Health Survey for England 2007: Healthy lifestyles: knowledge, attitudes and behaviour* Volume 1. London: The NHS Information Centre for Health and Social Care

Chellakooty M, Juul A, Boisen KA, Damgaard IN, Kai CM, Schmidt IM, Petersen JH, Skakkebaek NE, Main KM (2006) A prospective study of serum insulin-like growth factor I (IGF-I) and IGF-binding protein-3 in 942 healthy infants: associations with birth weight, gender, growth velocity, and breastfeeding. *J Clin Endocrinol Metab* 91: 820-826

Chinn S, Rona RJ (1984) The secular trend in the height of primary school children in England and Scotland from 1972-1980. *Ann Hum Biol* 11: 1-16

Clapp JF 3rd (2002) Maternal carbohydrate intake and pregnancy outcome. *Proc Nutr Soc* 61: 45-50

Cole TJ (1994) Do growth chart centiles need a face lift? *BMJ* 308: 641-642

Cole TJ (1995) Conditional reference charts to assess weight gain in British infants. *Arch Dis Child* 73(1): 8-16

Cole TJ (2000) Secular trends in growth. *Proc Nutr Soc* 59: 317-324

Cole TJ (2003) The secular trend in human physical growth: a biological view. *Econ Hum Biol* 1: 161-168

Cole TJ (2004a) Children grow and horses race: is the adiposity rebound a critical period for later obesity? *BMC Pediatr* 4: 6

Cole TJ (2004b) Modeling postnatal exposures and their interactions with birth size. *J Nutr* 134: 201-204

Cole TJ, Freeman JV, Preece AV (1998) British 1990 growth reference centiles for weight, height, body mass index and head circumference fitted by maximum penalized likelihood. *Statistics in Medicine* 17(4): 407-429

Cole ZA, Gale CR, Javaid MK, Robinson SM, Law C, Boucher BJ, Crozier SR, Godfrey KM, Dennison EM, Cooper C (2009) Maternal dietary patterns during pregnancy and childhood bone mass: a longitudinal study. *J Bone Miner Res* 24 (4): 663-668

Cole TJ, Paul AA, Whitehead RG (2002) Weight reference charts for British long-term breastfed infants. *Acta Paediatr* 91: 1296-1300

Condie R (1982) *Measurement of neonatal nutritional status in a multi-racial population. Nutrition in Pregnancy Symposium.* Royal College of Obstetrics and Gynaecology.

Constancia M, Angiolini E, Sandovici I, Smith P, Smith R, Kelsey G, Dean W, Ferguson-Smith A, Sibley CP, Reik W, Fowden A (2005) Adaptation of nutrient supply to fetal demand in the mouse involves interaction between the Igf2 gene and placental transporter systems. *Proc Natl Acad Sci USA* 102: 19219-19224

Conti J, Abraham S, Taylor A (1998) Eating behavior and pregnancy outcome. *J Psychosom Res* 44: 465-477

Cooney CA, Dave AA, Wolff GL (2002) Maternal methyl supplements in mice affect epigenetic variation and DNA methylation of offspring. *J Nutr* 132: S2393-S2400

Cooper C, Eriksson JG, Forsen T, Osmond C, Tuomilehto J, Barker DJ (2001) Maternal height, childhood growth and risk of hip fracture in later life: a longitudinal study. *Osteoporos Int* 12: 623-629

Cooper C, Javaid K, Westlake S, Harvey N, Dennison E (2005) Developmental origins of osteoporotic fracture: the role of maternal vitamin D insufficiency. *J Nutr* 135: S2728-S2734

Correa A, Gilboa SM, Besser LM, Botto LD, Moore CA, Hobbs CA, Cleves MA, Riehle-Colarusso TJ, Waller DK, Reece EA (2008) Diabetes mellitus and birth defects. *Am J Obs Gynecol* 199: 237

Coutinho, R, David, RJ, Collins JW Jr. (1997) Relation of parental birth weights to infant birth weight among African Americans and whites in Illinois: a transgenerational study. *Am J Epidemiol* 146(10): 804-809

Crowe C, Dandekar P, Fox M, Dhingra K, Bennet L, Hanson MA (1995) The effects of anaemia on heart, placenta and body weight, and blood pressure in fetal and neonatal rats. *J Physiol (Lond)* 488: 515-519

Crozier SR, Robinson SM, Godfrey KM, Cooper C, Inskip HM (2009) Women's dietary patterns change little from before to during pregnancy. *J Nutr* 139: 1956-1963

Dahri S, Snoeck A, Reusens-Billen B, Remacle C, Hoet JJ (1991) Islet function in offspring of mothers on low-protein diet during gestation. *Diabetes* 40(2): 115-120

Daniels SR, Morrison JA, Sprecher DL, Khoury P, Kimball TR (1999) Association of body fat distribution and cardiovascular risk factors in children and adolescents. *Circulation* 99: 541-545

Datta S, Alfaham M, Davies DP, Dunstan F, Woodhead S, Evans J, Richards B (2002) Vitamin D deficiency in pregnant women from a non-European ethnic minority population – an interventional study. *Br J Obstet Gynaecol* 109: 905-908

de Onis M, Blossner M, Villar J (1998) Levels and patterns of intrauterine growth retardation in developing countries. *Eur J Clin Nutr* 52 Suppl 1: S5-S15

De Stavola BL, dos Santos Silva I, McCormack V, Hardy RJ, Kuh DJ, Wadsworth ME (2004) Childhood growth and breast cancer. *Am J Epidemiol* 159: 671-682

de Weerd S, Steegers-Theunissen RP, de Boo TM, Thomas CM, Steegers EA (2003) Maternal periconceptional biochemical and hematological parameters, vitamin profiles and pregnancy outcome. *Eur J Clin Nutr* 57: 1128-1134

Dennison BA, Edmunds LS, Stratton HH, Pruzek RM (2006) Rapid infant weight gain predicts childhood overweight. *Obesity (Silver Spring)* 14: 491-499.

Department of Health (1991) *Dietary Reference Values for Food Energy and Nutrients for the United Kingdom*. Report on Health and Social Subjects 41. London: HMSO.

Department of Health (1994) *Weaning and the Weaning Diet*. Report on Health and Social Subjects 45. London: HMSO.

Department of Health (2000) *Folic acid and the prevention of disease*. Report on Health and Social Subjects 50. London: The Stationery Office.

Department of Health (2002) *Scientific Review of the Welfare Food Scheme*. Report on Health and Social Subjects 51. London: The Stationery Office.

Department of Health (2003) *Infant Feeding Recommendation*. Accessed online at: http://www.breastfeeding.nhs.uk/en/docs/FINAL_QA.pdf.

Department of Health (2008) *Healthy Start: Equality Impact Assessment*. Accessed online at: http://www.dh.gov.uk/en/Healthcare/Maternity/Maternalandinfantnutrition/DH_4112476

Desai M, Crowther NJ, Ozanne SE, Lucas A, Hales CN (1995) Adult glucose and lipid metabolism may be programmed during fetal life. *Biochem Soc Trans* 23(2): 331-335

Dewey KG, Peerson JM, Brown KH, Krebs NF, Michaelsen KF, Persson LA, Salmenpera L, Whitehead RG, Yeung DL (1995) Growth of breast-fed infants deviates from current reference data: a pooled analysis of US, Canadian, and European data sets. World Health Organization Working Group on Infant Growth. *Pediatrics* 96: 495-503

dos Santos Silva I, De Stavola BL, Hardy RJ, Kuh DJ, McCormack VA, Wadsworth ME (2004) Is the association of birth weight with premenopausal breast cancer risk mediated through childhood growth? *Br J Cancer* 91: 519-524

dos Santos Silva I, De Stavola B, McCormack V, Collaborative Group on Pre-natal Risk Factors and Subsequent Risk of Breast Cancer (2008) Birth size and breast cancer risk: re-analysis of individual participant data from 32 studies. *PLoS Med* 5(9): e193

Drake AJ, Walker BR (2004) The intergenerational effects of fetal programming: non-genomic mechanisms for the inheritance of low birth weight and cardiovascular risk. *J Endocrinol* 180: 1-16

Dubois L, Girard M (2006) Early determinants of overweight at 4.5 years in a population-based longitudinal study. *Int J Obes* 30: 610-617

Duggleby SL, Jackson AA (2002a) Higher weight at birth is related to decreased maternal amino acid oxidation during pregnancy. *Am J Clin Nutr* 76: 852-857

Duggleby SL, Jackson AA (2002b) Protein, amino acid and nitrogen metabolism during pregnancy: how might the mother meet the needs of her fetus? *Curr Opin Clin Nutr Metab Care* 5: 503-509

Edwards CR, Benediktsson R, Lindsay RS, Seckl JR (1993) Dysfunction of placental glucocorticoid barrier: link between fetal environment and adult hypertension? *Lancet* 341: 355-357

Egger M, Davey Smith G, Schneider M (2001) *Systematic reviews of observational studies.* In: *Systematic reviews in health care: Meta-analysis in context.* Egger M, Davey Smith G, Altman DG (eds). London: BMJ Publishing Group.

Ekbom A, Hsieh CC, Lipworth L, Wolk A, Ponten J, Adami HO, Trichopoulos D (1996) Perinatal characteristics in relation to incidence of and mortality from prostate cancer. *BMJ* 313: 337-341

Ekbom A, Wuu J, Adami HO, Lu CM, Lagiou P, Trichopoulos D, Hsieh CC (2000) Duration of gestation and prostate cancer risk in offspring. *Cancer Epidemiol Biomarkers Prev* 9: 221-223

Elia M, Betts P, Jackson DM, Mulligan J (2007) Fetal programming of body dimensions and percentage body fat measured in prepubertal children with a 4-component model of body composition, dual-energy X-ray absorptiometry, deuterium dilution, densitometry, and skinfold thicknesses. *Am J Clin Nutr* 86: 618-624

Elwood PC, Haley TJ, Hughes SJ, Sweetnam PM, Gray OP, Davies DP (1981) Child growth (0-5 years), and the effect of entitlement to a milk supplement. *Arch Dis Child* 56: 831-835

Engeland A, Bjorge T, Sogaard AJ, Tverdal A (2003) Body mass index in adolescence in relation to total mortality: 32-year follow-up of 227,000 Norwegian boys and girls. *Am J Epidemiol* 157: 517-523

Eriksson JG (2006) Early growth, and coronary heart disease and type 2 diabetes: experiences from the Helsinki Birth Cohort Studies. *Int J of Obesity* 30: S18-S22

Eriksson JG, Forsen T, Tuomilehto J, Osmond C, Barker DJ (2001) Early growth and coronary heart disease in later life: longitudinal study. *BMJ* 322: 949-953

Eriksson JG, Forsen T, Tuomilehto J, Osmond C, Barker DJ (2003) Early adiposity rebound in childhood and risk of type 2 diabetes in adult life. *Diabetologia* 46: 190-194

Eriksson JG, Forsen T, Tuomilehto J, Winter PD, Osmond C, Barker DJ (1999) Catch-up growth in childhood and death from coronary heart disease: longitudinal study. *BMJ* 318: 427-431

Eriksson JG, Lindi V, Uusitupa M, Forsen TJ, Laakso M, Osmond C, Barker DJP (2002) The effects of the Pro12Ala polymorphism of the peroxisome proliferator-activated receptor-$\gamma 2$ gene on insulin sensitivity and insulin metabolism interact with size at birth. *Diabetes* 51: 2321-2324

EURODIAB Substudy 2 Study Group (2002) Rapid early growth is associated with increased risk of childhood type 1 diabetes in various European populations. *Diabetes Care* 25: 1755-1760

Expert Group on Vitamins and Minerals (2003) *Safe Upper Levels for Vitamins and Minerals*. London: Food Standards Agency.

Fall C (1992) Nutrition in early life and later outcome. *Eur J Clin Nutr* 46 Suppl 4: S57-S63

Fall CH, Vijayakumar M, Barker DJ, Osmond C, Duggleby S (1995) Weight in infancy and prevalence of coronary heart disease in adult life. *BMJ* 310: 17-19

Finch S, Doyle W, Lowe C, Bates CJ, Prentice A, Smithers G, Clarke PC (1998) *National Diet and Nutrition Survey: people aged 65 years or over.* Volume 1: Report of the diet and nutrition survey. London: The Stationery Office.

Fisher D, Baird J, Payne L, Lucas P, Kleijnen J, Roberts H, Law C (2006) Are infant size and growth related to burden of disease in adulthood? A systematic review of literature. *Int J Epidemiol* 5: 1196-210

Floud R, Wachter K, Gregory A (1990) *Height, health and history: nutritional status in the United Kingdom, 1750-1980.* Cambridge: Cambridge University Press

Food and Agriculture Organization (2001) *Food and Nutrition Technical Report Series: Human energy requirements*. Report of a Joint FAO/WHO/UNU Expert Consultation, Rome. Accessed online at: ftp://ftp.fao.org/docrep/fao/007/y5686e/y5686e00.pdf.

Forman MR, Cantwell MM, Ronckers C, Zhang Y (2005) Through the looking glass at early-life exposures and breast cancer risk. *Cancer Invest* 23: 609-624

Forsdahl A (1977) Are poor living conditions in childhood and adolescence an important risk factor for arteriosclerotic heart disease? *Br J Prev Soc Med* 31: 91-95

Forsdahl A (1978) Living conditions in childhood and subsequent development of risk factors for arteriosclerotic heart disease. The cardiovascular survey in Finnmark 1974-75. *J Epidemiol Community Health* 32: 34-37

Forsen T, Eriksson J, Qiao Q, Tervahauta M, Nissinen A, Tuomilehto J (2000) Short stature and coronary heart disease: a 35-year follow-up of the Finnish cohorts of The Seven Countries Study. *J Intern Med* 248: 326-332

Forsen T, Eriksson JG, Tuomilehto J, Osmond C, Barker DJ (1999) Growth *in utero* and during childhood among women who develop coronary heart disease: longitudinal study. *BMJ* 319: 1403-1407

Forsen T, Eriksson JG, Tuomilehto J, Teramo K, Osmond C, Barker DJ (1997) Mother's weight in pregnancy and coronary heart disease in a cohort of Finnish men: follow up study. *BMJ* 315: 837-840

Foster K, Lader D, Cheesbrough S (1997) *Infant feeding 1995. A survey of infant feeding carried out by Social Survey Division of the ONS*. London: The Stationery Office.

Fraga MF, Ballestar E, Villar-Garea A, Boix-Chornet M, Espada J, Schotta G, Bonaldi T, Haydon C, Ropero S, Petrie K, Iyer NG, Perez-Rosado A, Calvo E, Lopez JA, Cano A, Calasanz MJ, Colomer D, Piris MA, Ahn N, Imhof A, Caldas C, Jenuwein T, Esteller M (2005). Loss of acetylation at Lys16 and trimethylation at Lys20 of histone H4 is a common hallmark of human cancer. *Nat Genet* 37: 391-400

Frankel S, Elwood P, Sweetnam P, Yarnell J, Davey Smith G (1996a) Birth weight, adult risk factors and incident coronary heart disease: the Caerphilly Study. *Public Health* 110: 139-143

Frankel S, Elwood P, Sweetnam P, Yarnell J, Davey Smith G (1996b) Birth weight, body-mass index in middle age, and incident coronary heart disease. *Lancet* 348: 1478-1480

Freeman AI, Munn HL, Lyons V, Dammermann A, Seckl JR, Chapman KE (2004) Glucocorticoid down-regulation of rat glucocorticoid receptor does not involve differential promoter regulation. *J Endocrinol* 183: 365-374

Gale CR, Ashurst HE, Hall NF, MacCallum PK, Martyn CN (2002) Size at birth and carotid atherosclerosis in later life. *Atherosclerosis* 163: 141-147

Gallou-Kabani C, Junien C (2005) Nutritional epigenomics of metabolic syndrome. *Diabetes* 54: 1899-1906

Gambling L, Andersen HS, Czopek A, Wojciak R, Krejpcio Z, McArdle HJ (2004) Effect of timing of iron supplementation on maternal and neonatal growth and iron status of iron-deficient pregnant rats. *J Physiol* 561: 195-203

Gambling L, Danzeisen R, Fosset C, Andersen HS, Dunford S, Srai SKS, McArdle HJ (2003) Iron and copper interactions in development and the effect on pregnancy outcome. *J Nutr* 133: S1-S3

Gamborg M, Byberg L, Rasmussen F, Andersen P, Baker JL, Bengtsson C, Canoy D, Droyvold W, Eriksson JG, Forsen T, Gunnarsdottir I, Jaqarvelin M, Koupil L, Lapidus L, Nilsen T, Olsen SF, Schack-Nielsen L, Thorsdottir I, Tuomainen T, Sorensen TIA (2007) Birth weight and systolic blood pressure in adolescence and adulthood: Meta-regression analysis of sex- and age-specific results from 20 nordic studies. *Am J Epidemiol* 166(6): 634-645

Ganpule A, Yajnik CS, Fall CH, Rao S, Fisher DJ, Kanade A, Cooper C, Naik S, Joshi N, Lubree H, Deshpande V, Joglekar C (2006) Bone mass in Indian children -relationships to maternal nutritional status and diet during pregnancy: the Pune Maternal Nutrition Study. *J Clin Endocrinol Metab.* 91(8): 2994-3001

Gardosi J, Chang A, Kalyan B, Sahota D, Symonds EM (1992) Customised antenatal growth charts. *Lancet* 339: 283-287

Garnica AD, Chan WY (1996) The role of the placenta in fetal nutrition and growth. *J Am Coll Nutr* 15: 206-222

Geleijnse JM, Hofman A, Witteman JCM, Hazebroek AAJM, Valkenburg HA, Grobbee DE (1997) Long-term effects of neonatal sodium restriction on blood pressure. *Hypertension* 29: 913-917

Gerstein HC (1994) Cow's milk exposure and type I diabetes mellitus. A critical overview of the clinical literature. *Diabetes Care* 17: 13-19

Gilbert JS, Lang AL, Grant AR, Nijland MJ (2005) Maternal nutrient restriction in sheep: hypertension and decreased nephron number in offspring at 9 months of age. *J Physiol* 565: 137-147

Gluckman PD, Hanson MA (2004) Maternal constraint of fetal growth and its consequences. In press Semin. *Fetal Neonat Med* 9: 419-425

Gluckman PD, Hanson MA, Buklijas T (2010) A conceptual framework for the developmental origins of health and disease. *Journal of Developmental Origins of Health and Disease* 1(1): 6-18

Gluckman PD, Hanson MA, Buklijas T, Low FM, Beedle AS (2009) Epigenetic mechanisms that underpin metabolic and cardiovascular diseases. *Nature Rev Endocrinol* 5: 401-408

Gnanalingham MG, Mostyn A, Dandrea J, Yakubu DP, Symonds ME, Stephenson T (2005) Ontogeny and nutritional programming of uncoupling protein-2 and glucocorticoid receptor mRNA in the ovine lung. *J Physiol* 565: 159-169

Godfrey KM (1998) Maternal regulation of fetal development and health in adult life. *Eur J Obstet Gynecol Reprod Biol* 78: 141-150

Godfrey KM, Barker DJ (2000) Fetal nutrition and adult disease. *Am J Clin Nutr* 71(5): S1344-S1352

Godfrey KM, Barker DJP, Peace J, Cloke J, Osmond C (1993) The relation of finger prints and the shape of the palm to patterns of fetal growth and adult blood pressure. *BMJ* 307: 405-409

Godfrey KM, Barker DJ, Robinson S, Osmond C (1997) Mother's birthweight and diet in pregnancy in relation to the baby's thinness at birth. *Br J Obstet Gynaecol* 104: 663-667

Godfrey KM, Redman CW, Barker DJ, Osmond C (1991) The effect of maternal anaemia and iron deficiency on the ratio of fetal weight to placental weight. *Br J Obstet Gynaecol* 98: 886-891

Godfrey K, Robinson S, Barker DJ, Osmond C, Cox V (1996) Maternal nutrition in early and late pregnancy in relation to placental and fetal growth. *BMJ* 312: 410-414

Goldbourt U, Tanne D (2002) Body height is associated with decreased long-term stroke but not coronary heart disease mortality? *Stroke* 33: 743-748

Goldenberg RL, Tamura T (1996) Prepregnancy weight and pregnancy outcome. *JAMA* 275: 1127-1128

Government Office for Science (2007) *Tackling obesity: future choices — summary of key messages*. London: Department for Innovation, Universities and Skills.

Graafmans WC, Richardus JH, Borsboom GJJM, Bakketeig L, Langhoff-Roos J, Bergsjo P, Macfarlane A, Verloove-Vanhorick SP, Mackenbach JP, EuroNatal working group (2002) Birth weight and perinatal mortality: a comparison of "optimal" birth weight in seven western european countries. *Epidemiology* 13(5): 569-574

Grainger RM, Hazard-Leonards RM, Samaha F, Hougan LM, Lesk MR, Thomsen GH (1983) Is hypomethylation linked to activation of delta-crystallin genes during lens development? *Nature* 306: 88-91

Green JR, Pawson IG, Schumacher LB, Perry J, Kretchmer N (1990) Glucose tolerance in pregnancy: ethnic variation and influence of body habitus. *Am J Obstet Gynecol* 163: 86-92

Gregory J, Collins DL, Davies PSW, Hughes JM, Clarke PC (1995) *National Diet and Nutrition Survey: Children aged 1½ to 4½ years*. Volume 1: Report of the diet and nutrition survey. London: HMSO.

Gregory J, Lowe S, Bates CJ, Prentice A, Jackson LV, Smithers G, Wenlock R, Farron M (2000) *National Diet and Nutrition Survey: young people aged 4 to 18 years*. Volume 1: Report of the diet and nutrition survey London: HMSO.

Gunnell D, Okasha M, Davey Smith G, Oliver SE, Sandhu J, Holly JMP (2001) Height, leg length, and cancer risk: a systematic review. *Epidemiol* Rev 23: 313-342

Gunnell DJ, Davey SG, Frankel S, Nanchahal K, Braddon FE, Pemberton J, Peters TJ (1998a) Childhood leg length and adult mortality: follow up of the Carnegie (Boyd Orr) Survey of Diet and Health in Pre-war Britain. *J Epidemiol Community Health* 52: 142-152

Gunnell DJ, Smith GD, Holly JMP, Frankel S (1998b) Leg length and risk of cancer in the Boyd Orr cohort. *BMJ* 317: 1350-1351

Guo SS, Chumlea WC (1999) Tracking of body mass index in children in relation to overweight in adulthood. *Am J Clin Nutr* 70: S145-S148

Haggarty P (2004) Effect of placental function on fatty acid requirements during pregnancy. *Eur J Clin Nutr* 58: 1559-1570

Haggarty P, Campbell DM, Duthie S, Andrews K, Hoad G, Piyathilake C, McNeill G (2009) Diet and deprivation in pregnancy. *Br J Nutr* 102: 1487-1497

Hales CN, Ozanne SE (2003) The dangerous road of catch-up growth. *J Physiol* 547: 5-10

Hall DMB, Elliman D (2003) *Health for all children*. Fourth edition. London: Oxford University Press.

Hamlyn B, Brooker S, Oleinikova K, Wands S (2002) *Infant feeding 2000: A survey conducted on behalf of the Department of Health, the Scottish Executive, the National Assembly for Wales and the Department of Health, Social Services and Public Safety in Northern Ireland*. London: The Stationery Office.

Hanson M, Gluckman P (2005) Endothelial dysfunction and cardiovascular disease: the role of predictive adaptive responses. *Heart* 91: 864-866

Harder T, Bergmann R, Kallischnigg G, Plagemann A (2005) Duration of breastfeeding and risk of overweight: a meta-analysis. *Am J Epidemiol* 162: 397-403

Harder T, Rodekamp E, Schellong K, Dudenhausen JW, Plagemann A (2007) Birth weight and subsequent risk of type 2 diabetes: a meta-analysis. *Am J Epidemiol* 165: 849-857

Harder T, Roepke K, Diller N, Stechling Y, Dudenhausen JW, Plagemann A (2009) Birth weight, early weight gain, and subsequent risk of type 1 diabetes: systematic review and meta-analysis. *Am J Epidemiol* 169(12): 1428-1436

Harding JE (2001) The nutritional basis of the fetal origins of adult disease. *Int J Epidemiol* 30: 15-23

Harding JE (2005) *Nutritional basis for the fetal origins of adult disease*. In: *Fetal nutrition and adult disease: programming of chronic disease through fetal exposure to undernutrition*, Langley-Evans SC (ed). Wallingford, Oxon: CABI.

Harding JE, McCowan LM (2003) Perinatal predictors of growth patterns to 18 months in children born small for gestational age. *Early Hum Dev* 74: 13-26

Harding S, Rosato MG, Cruickshank JK (2004) Lack of change in birthweights of infants by generational status among Indian, Pakistani, Bangladeshi, Black Caribbean, and Black African mothers in a British cohort study. *Int J Epidemiol* 33(6): 1279-1285

Hartung T (2008) Thoughts on limitations of animal studies. *Parkinsonism and Related Disorders* 14: S81-S83

Harvey NC, Javaid MK, Poole JR, Taylor P, Robinson SM, Inskip HM, Godfrey KM, Cooper C, Dennison EM: Southampton Women's Survey Study Group (2008) Paternal skeletal size predicts intrauterine bone mineral accrual. *J Clin Endocrinol Metab* 93: 1676-1681

Harvey NC, Robinson SM, Crozier SR, Marriott LD, Gale CR, Cole ZA, Inskip HM, Godfrey KM, Cooper C, Southampton Women's Survey Study Group (2009) Breast-feeding and adherence to infant feeding guidelines do not influence bone mass at age 4 years. *Br J Nutr* 102: 915-920

Haste FM, Brooke OG, Anderson HR, Bland JM (1991) The effect of nutritional intake on outcome of pregnancy in smokers and non-smokers. *Br J Nutr* 65: 347-354

Hawkesworth S (2009) Exploiting dietary supplementation trials to assess the impact of the prenatal environment on CVD risk. *Proc Nutr Soc* 68: 78-88

Hawkesworth S, Prentice AM, Fulford AJ, Moore SE (2008) Dietary supplementation of rural Gambian women during pregnancy does not affect body composition in offspring at 11-17 years of age. *J Nutr* 138: 2468-2473

Hawkesworth S, Prentice AM, Fulford AJC, Moore SE (2009) Maternal protein-energy supplementation does not affect adolescent blood pressure in the Gambia. *Int J Epidemiol* 38: 119-127

Hebert PR, Rich-Edwards JW, Manson JE, Ridker PM, Cook NR, O'Connor GT, Buring JE, Hennekens CH (1993) Height and incidence of cardiovascular disease in male physicians. *Circulation* 88: 1437-1443

Hediger ML, Overpeck MD, Ruan WJ, Troendle JF (2000) Early infant feeding and growth status of US-born infants and children aged 4-71 mo: analyses from the third National Health and Nutrition Examination Survey, 1988-1994. *Am J Clin Nutr* 72: 159-167

Heinig MJ, Nommsen LA, Peerson JM, Lonnerdal B, Dewey KG (1993) Energy and protein intakes of breast-fed and formula-fed infants during the first year of life and their association with growth velocity: the DARLING Study. *Am J Clin Nutr* 58: 152-161

Helland IB, Saugstad OD, Smith L, Saarem K, Solvoll K, Ganes T, Drevon CA (2001) Similar effects on infants of *n-3* and *n-6* fatty acids supplementation to pregnant and lactating women. *Pediatrics* 108: 82

Henderson L, Gregory J, Swan G (2002) *National Diet and Nutrition Survey: adults aged 19 to 64 years.* Volume 1: Types and quantities of foods consumed. London: The Stationery Office.

Henderson L, Gregory J, Irving K, Swan G (2003a) *National Diet and Nutrition Survey: adults aged 19 to 64 years*. Volume 2: Energy, protein, carbohydrate, fat and alcohol intake. London: The Stationery Office.

Henderson L, Irving K, Gregory J, Bates CJ, Prentice A, Perks J, Swan G, Farron M (2003b) *National Diet and Nutrition Survey: adults aged 19 to 64 years. Volume 3: Vitamin and mineral intake and urinary analytes*. London: The Stationery Office.

Herrera E (2000) Metabolic adaptations in pregnancy and their implications for the availability of substrates to the fetus. *Eur J Clin Nutr* 54 Suppl 1: S47-S51

Heslehurst N, Ells LJ, Simpson H, Batterham A, Wilkinson J, Summerbell C (2007) Trends in maternal obesity incidence rates, demographic predictors, and health inequalities in 36 821 women over a 15-year period. *Br J Obstet Gynaecol* 114: 187-194

Hilakivi-Clarke L, Forsen T, Eriksson JG, Luoto R, Tuomilehto J, Osmond C, Barker DJ (2001) Tallness and overweight during childhood have opposing effects on breast cancer risk. *Br J Cancer* 85: 1680-1684

Hillier TA, Pedula KL, Schmidt MM, Mullen JA, Charles MA, Pettitt DJ (2007) Childhood obesity and metabolic imprinting. The ongoing effects of maternal hyperglycemia. *Diabetes Care* 30: 2287-2292

Hiltunen MO, Turunen MP, Hakkinen TP, Rutanen J, Hedman M, Makinen K, Turunen AM, Aalto-Setala K, Yla-Herttuala S (2002) DNA hypomethylation and methyltransferase expression in atherosclerotic lesions. *Vasc Med* 7: 5-11

Hjalgrim LL, Rostgaard K, Hjalgrim H, Westergaard T, Thomassen H, Forestier E, Gustafsson G, Kristinsson J, Melbye M, Schmiegelow K (2004) Birth weight and risk for childhood leukemia in Denmark, Sweden, Norway, and Iceland. *J Natl Cancer Inst* 96: 1549-1556

Hjalgrim LL, Westergaard T, Rostgaard K, Schmiegelow K, Melbye M, Hjalgrim H, Engels EA (2003) Birth weight as a risk factor for childhood leukemia: a meta-analysis of 18 epidemiologic studies. *Am J Epidemiol* 158: 724-735

Hoddinott J, Maluccio JA, Behrman JR, Flores R, Martorell R (2008) Effect of a nutrition intervention in early childhood on economic productivity in Guatemalan adults. *Lancet* 371: 411-416

Hofman A, Hazebroek A, Valkenburg HA (1983) A randomized trial of sodium intake and blood pressure in newborn infants. *JAMA* 250: 370-373

Holick MF (2006) Resurrection of vitamin D deficiency and rickets. *J Clin Invest* 116: 2062-2072

Holness MJ, Langdown ML, Sugden MC (2000) Early-life programming of susceptibility to dysregulation of glucose metabolism and the development of Type 2 diabetes mellitus. *Biochemical Journal* 349: 657-665

Homko CJ, Sivan E, Reece EA, Boden G (1999) Fuel metabolism during pregnancy *Semin Reprod Endocrinol* 17: 119-125

Hoppe CC, Evans RG, Bertram JF, Moritz KM (2007) Effects of dietary protein restriction on nephron number in the mouse. *Am J Physiol Regul Integr Comp Physiol* 292: R1768-1774

Hoppe CC, Molgaard C, Michaelsen KF (2006) Cow's milk and linear growth in industrialized and developing countries. *Annu Rev Nutr* 26: 173

Horton TH (2005) Fetal origins of developmental plasticity: animal models of induced life history variation. *Am J Hum Biol* 17: 34-43

Horvath A, Koletzko B, Szajewska H (2007) Effect of supplementation of women in high-risk pregnancies with long-chain polyunsaturated fatty acids on pregnancy outcomes and growth measures at birth: a meta-analysis of randomized controlled trials. *Br J Nutr* 98: 253-259

Howie PW, Forsyth JS, Ogston SA, Clark A, Florey CD (1990) Protective effect of breastfeeding against infection. *BMJ* 300: 11-16

Huh SY, Rifas-Shiman SL, Kleinman KP, Rich-Edwards JW, Lipshultz SE, Gillman MW (2005) Maternal protein intake is not associated with infant blood pressure. *Int J Epidemiol* 34: 378-384

Huxley R, Neil A, Collins R (2002) Unravelling the fetal origins hypothesis: is there really an inverse association between birth weight and subsequent blood pressure? *Lancet* 360: 659-665

Huxley R, Owen CG, Whincup PH, Cook DG, Colman S, Collins R (2004) Birth weight and subsequent cholesterol levels: exploration of the "fetal origins" hypothesis. *JAMA* 292: 2755-2764

Huxley RR, Shiell AW, Law CM (2000) The role of size at birth and postnatal catch-up growth in determining systolic blood pressure: a systematic review of the literature. *J Hypertens* 18: 815-831

Huxley R, Owen CG, Whincup PH, Cook DG, Rich-Edwards J, Smith GD, Collins R (2007) Is birth weight a risk factor for ischemic heart disease in later life? *Am J Clin Nutr* 85: 1244-1250

Hypponen E, Leon DA, Kenward MG, Lithell H (2001) Prenatal growth and risk of occlusive and haemorrhagic stroke in Swedish men and women born 1915-29: historical cohort study. *BMJ* 323: 1033-1034

Hytten FE (1974) *Weight gain in pregnancy.* In: *Clinical Physiology in Obstetrics*, FE Hytten, JG Chamberlain (eds). Oxford: Blackwell Scientific Publications.

Ibanez L, Ong K, Dunger DB, de Zegher F (2006) Early development of adiposity and insulin resistance after catch-up weight gain in small-for-gestational-age children. *J Clin Endocrinol Metab* 91: 2153-2158

Inskip HM, Crozier SR, Godfrey KM, Borland SE, Cooper C, Robinson SM (2009) Women's compliance with nutrition and lifestyle recommendations before pregnancy: general population cohort study *BMJ* 12: 338-481

Ip S, Chung M, Raman G, Chew P, Magula N, DeVine D, Trikalinos T, Lau J (2007) *Breastfeeding and maternal and infant health outcomes in developed countries.* Evidence report/ Technology Assessment No 153. Rockville, MD: Agency for Healthcare Research and Quality.

Jackson AA (1996) *Perinatal nutrition: the impact on postnatal growth and development.* In: *Pediatrics and Perinataology,* Gluckman PD, Heymann MA (eds). London: Arnold

Jackson AA (2000) Nutrients, growth, and the development of programmed metabolic function. *Adv Exp Med Biol* 478: 41-55

Jackson AA (2005) Integrating the ideas of life course across cellular, individual, and population levels in cancer causation. *J Nutr* 135: S2927-S2933

Jackson AA, Bhutta ZA, Lumbiganon P (2003) Nutrition as a preventative strategy against adverse pregnancy outcomes. Introduction. *J Nutr* 133: S1589-S1591

Jackson AA, Dunn RL, Marchand MC, Langley-Evans SC (2002) Increased systolic blood pressure in rats induced by a maternal low-protein diet is reversed by dietary supplementation with glycine. *Clin Sci (Lond)* 103: 633-639

James DC (2001) Eating disorders, fertility, and pregnancy: relationships and complications. *J Perinat Neonatal Nurs* 15: 36-48

Jarjou LM, Prentice A, Sawo Y, Laskey MA, Bennett J, Goldberg GR, Cole TJ (2006) Randomized, placebo-controlled, calcium supplementation study in pregnant Gambian women: effects on breast-milk calcium concentrations and infant birth weight, growth, and bone mineral accretion in the first year of life *Am J Clin Nutr* 83 (3): 657-666

Javaid MK, Crozier SR, Harvey NC, Gale CR, Dennison EM, Boucher BJ, Arden NK, Godfrey KM, Cooper C (2006) Maternal vitamin D status during pregnancy and childhood bone mass at age 9 years: a longitudinal study. *Lancet* 367: 36-43

Jones RL, Cederberg HMS, Wheeler SJ, Poston L, Hutchinson CJ, Seed PT, Oliver RL, Baker PN (2009) Relationship between maternal growth, infant birthweight and nutrient partitioning in teenage pregnancies. *Br J Obstet Gynaecol* 117(2): 200-211

Joseph KS, Kramer MS (1996) Review of the evidence on fetal and early childhood antecedents of adult chronic disease. *Epidemiol Rev* 18: 158-174

Joshi NP, Kulkarni SR, Yajnik CS, Joglekar CV, Rao S, Coyaji KJ, Lubree HG, Rege SS, Fall CH (2005) Increasing maternal parity predicts neonatal adiposity: Pune Maternal Nutrition Study. *Am J Obstet Gynecol* 193: 783-789

Jousilahti P, Tuomilehto J, Vartiainen E, Eriksson J, Puska P (2000) Relation of adult height to cause-specific and total mortality: a prospective follow-up study of 31,199 middle-aged men and women in Finland. *Am J Epidemiol* 151: 1112-1120

Jovanovic-Peterson L, Peterson CM, Reed GF, Metzger BE, Mills JL, Knopp RH, Aarons JH (1991) Maternal postprandial glucose levels and infant birth weight: the Diabetes in Early Pregnancy Study. The National Institute of Child Health and Human Development-Diabetes in Early Pregnancy Study. *Am J Obstet Gynecol* 164: 103-111

Kahn HS, Graff M, Stein AD, Lumey LH (2009) A fingerprint marker from early gestation associated with diabetes in middle age: The Dutch Hunger Winter Families Study. *Int J Epidemiol*. 38(1): 101-109

Kahn HS, Graff M, Stein AD, Zybert PA, Mckeague IW, Lumey LH (2008) A fingerprint characteristic associated with the early prenatal environment. *Am J Human Biology* 20: 59-65

Kaijser M, Akre O, Cnattingius S, Ekbom A (2005) Preterm birth, low birth weight, and risk for esophageal adenocarcinoma. *Gastroenterology* 128: 607-609

Kajantie E, Osmond C, Barker DJ, Forsen T, Phillips DI, Eriksson JG (2005) Size at birth as a predictor of mortality in adulthood: a follow-up of 350 000 person-years. *Int J Epidemiol* 34: 655-663

Karaolis-Danckert N, Buyken AE, Bolzenius K, Perim de Faria C, Lentze MJ, Kroke A (2006) Rapid growth among term children whose birth weight was appropriate for gestational age has a longer lasting effect on body fat percentage than on body mass index. *Am J Clin Nutr* 84: 1449-1455

Karlberg J (1989) A biologically-oriented mathematical model (ICP) for human growth. *Acta Paediatr Scand* Suppl 350. 70 94

Karlberg J, Jalil F, Lam B, Low L, Yeung CY (1994) Linear growth retardation in relation to the three phases of growth. *Eur J Clin Nutr* 48 Suppl 1: S25-S43; Discussion S43-4

Kelly Y, Panico L, Bartley M, Marmot M, Nazroo J, Sacker A (2008) Why does birthweight vary among ethnic groups in the UK? Findings from the Millennium Cohort Study. *J Public Health Med* 31(1): 131-137

Kensara OA, Wootton SA, Phillips DI, Patel M, Hoffman DJ, Jackson AA, Elia M (2006) Substrate-energy metabolism and metabolic risk factors for cardiovascular disease in relation to fetal growth and adult body composition. *Am J Physiol Endocrinol Metab* 291: E365-E371

Kensara OA, Wootton SA, Phillips DI, Patel M, Jackson AA, Elia M (2005) Fetal programming of body composition: relation between birth weight and body composition measured with dual-energy X-ray absorptiometry and anthropometric methods in older Englishmen. *Am J Clin Nutr* 82: 980-987

Kinra S, Rameshwar Sarma KV, Ghafoorunissa, Mendu VV, Ravikumar R, Mohan V, Wilkinson IB, Cockcroft JR, Davey Smith G, Ben-Shlomo Y (2008) Effect of integration of supplemental nutrition with public health programmes in pregnancy and early childhood on cardiovascular risk in rural Indian adolescents: long term follow-up of Hyderabad nutrition trial. *BMJ* 337: 1-10

Knopp RH (1997) Hormone-mediated changes in nutrient metabolism in pregnancy: a physiological basis for normal fetal development. *Ann N Y Acad Sci* 817: 251-271

Koletzko B, Broekaert I, Demmelmair H, Franke J, Hannibal I, Oberle D, Schiess S, Baumann BT, Verwied-Jorky S (2005) Protein intake in the first year of life: a risk factor for later obesity? The EU childhood obesity project. *Adv Exp Med Biol.* 569: 69-79.

Koletzko B, von Kries R, Closa R, Escribano J, Scaglioni S, Giovannini M, Beyer J, Demmelmair H, Anton B, Gruszfeld D, Dobrzanska A, Sengier A, Langhendries JP, Rolland Cachera MF, Grote V (2009a) Can infant feeding choices modulate later obesity risk? *Am J Clin Nutr* 89(5): S1502-S1508

Koletzko B, von Kries R, Closa R, Escribano J, Scaglioni S, Giovannini M, Beyer J, Demmelmair H, Gruszfeld D, Dobrzanska A, Sengier A, Langhendries JP, Rolland Cachera MF, Grote V (2009b) Lower protein in infant formula is associated with lower weight up to age 2 y: a randomized clinical trial. *Am J Clin Nutr* 89(6): 1836-1845

Koprowski C, Ross RK, Mack WJ, Henderson BE, Bernstein L (1999) Diet, body size and menarche in a multiethnic cohort. *Br J Cancer* 79: 1907-1911

Koupilova I, Leon DA, McKeigue PM, Lithell HO (1999) Is the effect of low birth weight on cardiovascular mortality mediated through high blood pressure? *J Hypertens* 17: 19-25

Kramer MS (1987) Determinants of low birth weight: methodological assessment and meta-analysis. *Bull World Health Organ* 65: 663-737

Kramer MS (2003) The epidemiology of adverse pregnancy outcomes: an overview. *J Nutr* 133: S1592-S1596

Kramer MS, Chalmers B, Hodnett ED, Sevkovskaya Z, Dzikovich I, Shapiro S, Collet JP, Vanilovich I, Mezen I, Ducruet T, Shishko G, Zubovich V, Mknuik D, Gluchanina E, Dombrovskiy V, Ustinovitch A, Kot T, Bogdanovich N, Ovchinikova L, Helsing E (2001) Promotion of Breastfeeding Intervention Trial (PROBIT): a randomized trial in the Republic of Belarus. *JAMA* 285: 413-420

Kramer MS, Guo T, Platt RW, Shapiro S, Collet JP, Chalmers B, Hodnett E, Sevkovskaya Z, Dzikovich I, Vanilovich I (2002) Breastfeeding and infant growth: biology or bias? *Pediatrics* 110: 343-347

Kramer MS, Guo T, Platt RW, Vanilovich I, Sevkovskaya Z, Dzikovich I, Michaelsen KF, Dewey K (2004) Feeding effects on growth during infancy. *J Pediatr* 145: 600-605

Kramer S, Kakuma R (2002) *The optimal duration of exclusive feeding: A systematic review.* Cochrane Database Syst Rev 1, CD003517

Kramer MS, Kakuma R (2003) *Energy and protein intake in pregnancy.* Cochrane Database Syst Rev 4, CD000032

Kramer MS, Matush L, Vanilovich I, Platt RW, Bogdanovich N, Sevkovskaya Z, Dzikovich I, Shishko G, Collet JP, Martin RM, Davey Smith G, Gillman MW, Chalmers B, Hodnett E, Shapiro S, for the Promotion of Breastfeeding Intervention Trial (PROBIT) Study Group

(2007) Effects of prolonged and exclusive breastfeeding on child height, weight, adiposity, and blood pressure at age 6.5 y: evidence from a large randomized trial. *Am J Clin Nutr* 86: 1717-1721

Kramer MS, McLean FH, Olivier M, Willis DM, Usher RH (1989) Body proportionality and head and length 'sparing' in growth-retarded neonates: a critical reappraisal. *Pediatrics* 84: 717-723

Kramer MS, Victora CG (2001) *Low birth weight and perinatal mortality.* In: *Nutrition and Health in Developing Countries.* Semba RD, Bloem MW (eds). Totowa, NJ: Humana Press

Kristensen J, Vestergaard M, Wisborg K, Kesmodel U, Secher NJ (2005) Pre-pregnancy weight and the risk of stillbirth and neonatal death. *Br J Obstet Gynaecol* 112: 403-408

Kuh DL, Power C, Rodgers B (1991) Secular trends in social class and sex differences in adult height. *Int J Epidemiol* 20: 1001-1009

Langer O, Yogev Y, Xenakis EM, Brustman L (2005) Overweight and obese in gestational diabetes: the impact on pregnancy outcome. *Am J Obstet Gynecol* 192: 1768-1776

Langley SC, Jackson AA (1994) Increased systolic pressure in adult rats induced by fetal exposure to maternal low protein diet. *Clin Sci* 86: 217-222

Langley SC, Browne RF, Jackson AA (1994) Altered glucose tolerance in rats exposed to maternal low protein diets *in utero. Comp Biochem Physiol* 109: 223-229

Langley Evans SC (2001) Fetal programming of cardiovascular function through exposure to maternal undernutrition. *Proc Nutr Soc* 60: 505-513

Langley-Evans SC (2004) *Fetal nutrition and adult disease: programming of chronic disease through fetal exposure to undernutrition.* Wallingford, Oxon: CABI Publishing.

Langley-Evans SC (2006) Developmental programming of health and disease. *Proc Nutr Soc* 65: 97-105

Langley-Evans SC, Phillips GJ, Benediktsson R, Gardner DS, Edwards CR, Jackson AA, Seckl JR (1996) Protein intake in pregnancy, placental glucocorticoid metabolism and the programming of hypertension in the rat. *Placenta* 17: 169-172

Langley-Evans SC, Welham SJ, Jackson AA (1999) Fetal exposure to a maternal low protein diet impairs nephrogenesis and promotes hypertension in the rat. *Life Sci* 64: 965-974

Larnkjaer A, Schroder SA, Schmidt IM, Jorgensen MH, Michaelsen KF (2006) Secular change in adult stature has come to a halt in northern Europe and Italy. *Acta Paediatrica* 95: 754-755

Lashen H, Fear K, Sturdee DW (2004) Obesity is associated with increased risk of first trimester and recurrent miscarriage: matched case control study. *Hum Reprod* 19: 1644-1646

Lauren L, Jarvelin MR, Elliott P, Sovio U, Spellman A, McCarthy M, Emmett P, Rogers I, Hartikainen AL, Pouta A, Hardy R, Wadsworth M, Helmsdal G, Olsen S, Bakoula C, Lekea V, Millwood I (2003) Relationship between birth weight and blood lipid concentrations in later life: evidence from the existing literature. *Int J Epidemiol* 32: 862-876

Law CM, de Swiet M, Osmond C, Fayers PM, Barker DJ, Cruddas AM, Fall CH (1993) Initiation of hypertension *in utero* and its amplification throughout life. *BMJ* 306: 24-27

Law CM, Shiell AW (1996) Is blood pressure inversely related to birth weight? The strength of evidence from a systematic review of the literature. *J Hypertens* 14: 935-941

Lawlor DA, Owen CG, Davies AA, Whincup PH, Ebrahim S, Cook DG, Davey SG (2006) Sex differences in the association between birth weight and total cholesterol. A meta-analysis. *Ann Epidemiol* 16: 19-25

Lawlor DA, Riddoch CJ, Page AS, Andersen LB, Wedderkopp N, Harro M, Stansbie D, Smith GD (2005) Infant feeding and components of the metabolic syndrome: findings from the European Youth Heart Study. *Arch Dis Child* 90: 582-588

Le Marchand L, Kolonel LN, Earle ME, Mi MP (1988) Body size at different periods of life and breast cancer risk. *Am J Epidemiol* 128: 137-152

Lenders CM, Hediger ML, Scholl TO, Khoo CS, Slap GB, Stallings VA (1994) Effect of high-sugar intake by low-income pregnant adolescents on infant birth weight. *J Adolesc Health* 15: 596-602

Leon DA, Lithell HO, Vagero D, Koupilova I, Mohsen R, Berglund L, Lithell UB, McKeigue PM (1998) Reduced fetal growth rate and increased risk of death from ischaemic heart disease: cohort study of 15 000 Swedish men and women born 1915-29. *BMJ* 317: 241-245

Lewis G (2007) Saving Mothers Lives. *The seventh report of the UK confidential enquires into maternal deaths 2000-02.* London: CEMACH.

Lewis RM, Doherty CB, James LA, Burton GJ, Hales CN (2001) Effects of maternal iron restriction on placental vascularization in the rat. *Placenta* 22: 534-539

Li H, Stein AD, Barnhart HX, Ramakrishnan U, Martorell R (2003) Associations between prenatal and postnatal growth and adult body size and composition. *Am J Clinical Nutr* 77: 1498-1505

Lillycrop KA, Phillips ES, Jackson AA, Hanson MA, Burdge GC (2005) Dietary protein restriction of pregnant rats induces and folic acid supplementation prevents epigenetic modification of hepatic gene expression in the offspring. *J Nutr* 135: 1382-1386

Lillycrop KA, Slater-Jefferies JL, Hanson MA, Godfrey KM, Jackson AA, Burdge GC (2007) Induction of altered epigenetic regulation of the hepatic glucocorticoid receptor in the offspring of rats fed a protein-restricted diet during pregnancy suggests that reduced DNA methyltransferase-1 expression is involved in impaired DNA methylation and changes in histone modifications. *Br J Nutr* 97: 1064-1073

Lisle SJ, Lewis RM, Petry CJ, Ozanne SE, Hales CN, Forhead AJ (2003) Effect of maternal iron restriction during pregnancy on renal morphology in the adult rat offspring. *Brit J Nutr* 90: 33-39

Little RE, Wendt JK (1991) The effects of maternal drinking in the reproductive period: an epidemiologic review. *J Subst Abuse* 3: 187-204

Liu L, Li Y, Tollefisbol TO (2008) Gene-environment interactions and epigenetic basis of human diseases. *Curr Issues Mol Biol* 10: 25-36

Locker J, Reddy TV, Lombardi B (1986) DNA methylation and hepatocarcinogenesis in rats fed a choline-devoid diet. *Carcinogenesis* 7: 1309-1312

Loos RJ, Beunen G, Fagard R, Derom C, Vlietinck R (2001) Birth weight and body composition in young adult men – a prospective twin study. *Int J Obes Relat Metab Disord* 25: 1537-1545

Lopuhaa CE, Roseboom TJ, Osmond C, Barker DJ, Ravelli AC, Bleker OP, van der Zee JS, van der Meulen JH (2000) Atopy, lung function, and obstructive airways disease after prenatal exposure to famine. *Thorax* 55: 555-561

Lucas A (1991) *Programming by early nutrition in man*. In: *The Childhood Environment and Adult Disease*, Bock GR, Whelan J (eds). Chichester, West Sussex: John Wiley and Sons.

Lucas A (1994) Role of nutritional programming in determining adult morbidity. *Arch Dis Child* 71. 288-290

Lucas A (1998) Programming by early nutrition: an experimental approach. *J Nutr* 128(2): S401-S406

Lucas A, Fewtrell MS, Cole TJ (1999) Fetal origins of adult disease – the hypothesis revisited. *BMJ* 319: 245-249

Ludvigsson JF, Ludvigsson J (2004) Milk consumption during pregnancy and infant birth weight. *Acta Paediatr* 93: 1474-1478

Lumey LH (1992) Decreased birth weights in infants after maternal *in utero* exposure to the Dutch famine of 1944-1945. *Paediatr Perinat Epidemiol* 6: 240-253

Lumey LH, Ravelli AC, Wiessing LG, Koppe JG, Treffers PE, Stein ZA (1993) The Dutch famine birth cohort study: design, validation of exposure, and selected characteristics of subjects after 43 years follow-up. *Paediatr Perinat Epidemiol* 7: 354-367

Lumley J, Oliver S, Waters E (2000) *Interventions for promoting smoking cessation during pregnancy*. Cochrane Database Syst Rev 3, CD001055

Lumley J, Oliver S, Chamberlain C, Oakley L (1998) *Interventions for promoting smoking cessation during pregnancy*. Cochrane Database of Syst Rev 3, CD001055

Lund G, Andersson L, Lauria M, Lindholm M, Fraga MF, Villar-Garea A, Ballestar E, Esteller M, Zaina S (2004) DNA methylation polymorphisms precede any histological sign of atherosclerosis in mice lacking apolipoprotein E. *J Biol Chem* 279: 29147-29154

Malcolm CA, Hamilton R, McCulloch DL, Montgomery C, Weaver LT (2003) Scotopic electroretinogram in term infants born of mothers supplemented with docosahexaenoic acid during pregnancy. *Invest Ophthalmol Vis Sci* 44: 3685-3691

Maloney CA, Gosby AK, Phuyal JL, Denyer GS, Bryson JM, Caterson ID (2003) Site-specific changes in the expression of fat-partitioning genes in weanling rats exposed to a low-protein diet *in utero*. *Obes Res* 11: 461-468

Mannion CA, Gray-Donald K, Koski KG (2006) Association of low intake of milk and vitamin D during pregnancy with decreased birth weight. *CMAJ* 174: 1273-1277

Marchand MC, Langley-Evans SC (2001) Intrauterine programming of nephron number: the fetal flaw revisited. *J Nephrol* 14: 327-331

Margetts BM, Mohd Yusof S, Al Dallal Z, Jackson AA (2002) Persistence of lower birth weight in second generation South Asian babies born in the United Kingdom. *J Epidemiol Community Health* 56: 684-687

Marmot MG (1984) Geography of blood pressure and hypertension. *Br Med Bull* 40: 380-386

Marmot MG, Page CM, Atkins E, Douglas JW (1980) Effect of breast-feeding on plasma cholesterol and weight in young adults. *J Epidemiol Community Health* 34: 164-167

Marmot MG, Shipley MJ, Rose G (1984) Inequalities in death — specific explanations of a general pattern? *Lancet* 1: 1003-1006

Martin RM, Davey Smith G, Mangtani P, Frankel S, Gunnell D (2002) Association between breast feeding and growth: the Boyd-Orr cohort study. *Arch Dis Child Fetal Neonatal Ed* 87: F193-F201

Martin RM, Gunnell D, Owen CG, Smith GD (2005a) Breast-feeding and childhood cancer: A systematic review with metaanalysis. *Int J Cancer* 117: 1020-1031

Martin RM, Gunnell D, Smith GD (2005b) Breastfeeding in infancy and blood pressure in later life: systematic review and meta-analysis. *Am J Epidemiol* 161: 15-26

Martin RM, Holly JM, Davey Smith G, Ness AR, Emmett P, Rogers I, Gunnell D (2005c) Could associations between breastfeeding and insulin-like growth factors underlie associations of breastfeeding with adult chronic disease? The Avon Longitudinal Study of Parents and Children. *Clin Endocrinol (Oxf)* 62: 728-737

Martin RM, Middleton N, Gunnell D, Owen CG, Smith GD (2005d) Breast-feeding and cancer: the Boyd Orr cohort and a systematic review with meta-analysis. *J Natl Cancer Inst* 97: 1446-1457

Martin RM, Ness AR, Gunnell D, Emmett P, Davey SG (2004b) Does breast-feeding in infancy lower blood pressure in childhood? The Avon Longitudinal Study of Parents and Children (ALSPAC). *Circulation* 109: 1259-1266

Martin RM, Smitha GD, Mangtanib P, Tillinga K, Frankela S, Gunnella D (2004a) Breastfeeding and cardiovascular mortality: the Boyd Orr cohort and a systematic review with meta-analysis. *Eur Heart J* 25: 778-786

Martyn CN, Gale CR, Jespersen S, Sherriff SB (1998) Impaired fetal growth and atherosclerosis of carotid and peripheral arteries. *Lancet* 352: 173-178

Mathews F, Neil HAW (1998) Nutrient intakes during pregnancy in a cohort of nulliparous women. *J Hum Nutr Diet* 11: 151-161

McCarron P, Okasha M, McEwen J, Davey Smith G (2002) Height in young adulthood and risk of death from cardiorespiratory disease: a prospective study of male former students of Glasgow University, Scotland. *Am J Epidemiol* 155: 683-687

McCarthy A, Hughes R, Tilling K, Davies D, Davey Smith G, Ben Shlomo Y (2007) Birth weight; postnatal, infant, and childhood growth; and obesity in young adulthood: evidence from the Barry Caerphilly Growth Study. *Am J Clin Nutr* 86: 907-913

McCormack VA, dos Santos Silva I, Koupil I, Leon DA, Lithell HO (2005) Birth characteristics and adult cancer incidence: Swedish cohort of over 11,000 men and women. *Int J Cancer* 115: 611-617

McGarvey SI, Zinner SH, Willett WC, Rosner B (1991) Maternal prenatal dietary potassium, calcium, magnesium, and infant blood pressure. *Hypertension* 17: 218-224

McGrath JJ, Keeping D, Saha S, Chant DC, Lieberman DE, O'Callaghan MJ (2005) Seasonal fluctuations in birth weight and neonatal limb length; does prenatal vitamin D influence neonatal size and shape? *Early Hum Dev* 81: 609-618

McMullen S, Mostyn A (2009) Animal models for the study of the developmental origins of health and disease. *Proc Nutr Soc* 68: 1-15

Mehta KC, Specker B, Bartholmey S, Giddens J, Ho LM (1998) Trial on timing of introduction to solids and food type on infant growth. *Pediatrics* 102: 569-573

Mei Z, Grummer-Strawn LM, Thompson D, Dietz WH (2004) Shifts in percentiles of growth during early childhood: analysis of longitudinal data from the California Child Health and Development Study. *Pediatrics* 113: e617-e627

Metcalfe NB, Monaghan P (2001) Compensation for a bad start: grow now, pay later? *Trends in Ecology and Evolution* 16(5): 254-260

Milne E, Laurvick CL, Blair E, Bower C, de Klerk N (2007) Fetal growth and acute childhood leukemia: looking beyond birth weight. *Am J Epidemiol* 166: 151-159

Mitchell EA, Robinson E, Clark PM, Becroft DM, Glavish N, Pattison NS, Pryor JE, Thompson JM, Wild CJ (2004) Maternal nutritional risk factors for small for gestational age babies in a developed country: a case-control study. *Arch Dis Child Fetal Neonatal Ed* 89: F431-F435

Moisan J, Meyer F, Gingras S (1990) Diet and age at menarche. *Cancer Causes Control* 1: 149-154

Monteiro PO, Victora CG (2005) Rapid growth in infancy and childhood and obesity in later life: a systematic review. *Obes Rev* 6: 143-154

Moore VM, Davies MJ, Willson KJ, Worsley A, Robinson JS (2004) Dietary composition of pregnant women is related to size of the baby at birth. *J Nutr* 134: 1820-1826

Moran VH (2007) A systematic review of dietary assessments of pregnant adolescents in industrialised countries. *Br J Nutr* 97: 411-425

Morgan JB, Lucas A, Fewtrell MS (2004) Does weaning influence growth and health up to 18 months? *Arch Dis Child* 89: 728-733

Morley R, Lucas A (2000) Randomized diet in the neonatal period and growth performance until 7.5–8 y of age in preterm children *Am J Clin Nut* 71: 822-828

Morrison J, Williams GM, Najman JM, Andersen MJ (1991) The influence of paternal height and weight on birthweight. *Aust N Z J Obstet Gynaecol* 31: 114-116

Moses RG, Luebcke M, Davis WS, Coleman KJ, Tapsell LC, Petocz P, Brand-Miller JC (2006) Effect of a low-glycemic-index diet during pregnancy on obstetric outcomes. *Am J Clin Nutr* 84: 807-812

Mouratidou T, Ford F, Prountzou F, Fraser R (2006) Dietary assessment of a population of pregnant women in Sheffield, UK. *Br J Nutr* 96: 929-935

Murphy JF, O'Riordan J, Newcombe RG, Coles EC, Pearson JF (1986) Relation of haemoglobin levels in first and second trimester to outcome of pregnancy. *Lancet* 1: 992-994

Murphy VE, Smith R, Giles WB, Clifton VL (2006) Endocrine regulation of human fetal growth: the role of the mother, placenta, and fetus. *Endocrin Rev* 27(2): 141-169

Myles TD, Gooch J, Santolaya J (2002) Obesity is an independent risk factor for infectious morbidity in patients who undergo caesarean delivery. *Obstet Gynecol* 100: 959-964

National Institute for Health and Clinical Excellence (2008a) *Improving the nutrition of pregnant and breastfeeding mothers and children in low-income households*. NICE Public Health Guideline 11.

National Institute for Health and Clinical Excellence (2008b) *Antenatal Care: Routine care for the healthy pregnant woman*. NICE Clinical Guideline 62.

National Institute for Health and Clinical Excellence (2010) *Dietary interventions and physical activity interventions for weight management before, during and after pregnancy*. NICE Public Health Guideline 27.

National Perinatal Epidemiology Unit (2007) *Preliminary results from the extreme obesity in pregnancy survey in the UK*. UKOSS. Accessed online at: www.npeu.ox.ac.uk

Nelson M, Erens B, Bates B, Church S, Boshier T (2007) *Low Income Diet and Nutrition Survey*. London: The Stationery Office.

Newsome CA, Shiell AW, Fall CH, Phillips DI, Shier R, Law CM (2003) Is birth weight related to later glucose and insulin metabolism? A systematic review. *Diabetic Medicine* 20: 339-348

Nilsen TI, Romundstad PR, Troisi R, Potischman N, Vatten LJ (2005a) Birth size and colorectal cancer risk: a prospective population based study. *Gut* 54: 1728-1732

Nilsen TI, Romundstad PR, Troisi R, Vatten LJ (2005b) Birth size and subsequent risk for prostate cancer: a prospective population-based study in Norway. *Int J Cancer* 113: 1002-1004

Norris JM, Scott FW (1996) A meta-analysis of infant diet and insulin-dependent diabetes mellitus: do biases play a role? *Epidemiology* 7: 87-92

Office for National Statistics (2000) *Birth Statistics. Review of the Registrar General on Births and Patterns of Family Building in England and Wales*. Series FM1 no. 29. London: Office for National Statistics.

Ohmi H, Hirooka K, Hata A, Mochizuki Y (2001) Recent trend of increase in proportion of low birth weight infants in Japan. *Int J Epidemiol* 30: 1269-1271

Okasha M, McCarron P, Gunnell D, Smith GD (2003) Exposures in childhood, adolescence and early adulthood and breast cancer risk: a systematic review of the literature. *Breast Cancer Res Treat* 78: 223-276

Olausson H, Laskey MA, Goldberg GR, Prentice A (2008) Changes in bone mineral status and bone size during pregnancy and the influences of body weight and calcium intake. *Am J Clin Nutr* 88: 1032-1039

Olsen SF, Halldorsson TI, Willett WC, Knudsen VK, Gillman MW, Mikkelsen TB, Olsen J, The NUTRIX Consortium (2007) Milk consumption during pregnancy is associated with increased infant size at birth: prospective cohort study. *Am J Clin Nutr* 86: 1104-1110

Olsen SF, Secher NJ, Tabor A, Weber T, Walker JJ, Gluud C (2000) Randomised clinical trials of fish oil supplementation in high risk pregnancies. Fish Oil Trials In Pregnancy (FOTIP) Team. *Br J Obstet Gynaecol* 107: 382-395

Olsen SF, Sorensen JD, Secher NJ, Hedegaard M, Henriksen TB, Hansen HS, Grant A (1992) Randomised controlled trial of effect of fish-oil supplementation on pregnancy duration. *Lancet* 339: 1003-1007

Ong KK, Ahmed ML, Emmett PM, Preece MA, Dunger DB (2000) Association between postnatal catch-up growth and obesity in childhood: prospective cohort study. *BMJ* 320: 967-971

Ong KK, Loos RJ (2006) Rapid infancy weight gain and subsequent obesity: systematic reviews and hopeful suggestions. *Acta Paediatr* 95: 904-908

Ong KK, Northstone K, Wells JC, Rubin C, Ness AR (2007) Earlier mother's age at menarche predicts rapid infancy growth and childhood obesity. *PLoS Med* 4(4): e132

Onland-Moret NC, Peeters PH, van Gils CH, Clavel-Chapelon F, Key T, Tjønneland A, Trichopoulou A, Kaaks R, Manjer J, Panico S, Palli D, Tehard B, Stoikidou M, Bueno-De-Mesquita HB, Boeing H, Overvad K, Lenner P, Quirós JR, Chirlaque MD, Miller AB, Khaw KT, Riboli E (2005) Age at menarche in relation to adult height: The EPIC study. *Am J Epidemiol* 162: 623-632

Oppe TE (1974) *Present-day practice in infant feeding report of a working party of the Panel on Child Nutrition*, Committee on Medical Aspects of Food Policy. London: HMSO.

Oppe TE (1980) *Artificial feeds for the young infant report of the Working Party on the Composition of Foods for Infants and Young Children*, Committee on Medical Aspects of Food Policy. London: HMSO.

Osmond C, Barker DJ, Winter PD, Fall CH, Simmonds SJ (1993) Early growth and death from cardiovascular disease in women. *BMJ* 307: 1519-1524

Owen CG, Martin RM, Whincup PH, Smith GD, Cook DG (2005) Effect of infant feeding on the risk of obesity across the life course: a quantitative review of published evidence. *Pediatrics* 115: 1367-1377

Owen CG, Martin RM, Whincup PH, Smith GD, Cook DG (2006) Does breastfeeding influence risk of type 2 diabetes in later life? A quantitative analysis of published evidence. *Am J Clin Nutr* 84: 1043-1054

Owen CG, Nightingale CM, Rudnicka AR, Cook DG, Ekelund U, Whincup PH (2009a) Ethnic and gender differences in physical activity levels among 9-10-year-old children of white European, South Asian and African-Caribbean origin: the Child Heart Health Study in England (CHASE Study). *Int J Epidemiol* 38: 1082-1093

Owen CG, Whincup PH, Gilg JA, Cook DG (2003a) Effect of breast feeding in infancy on blood pressure in later life: systematic review and meta-analysis. *BMJ* 327: 1189-1195

Owen CG, Whincup PH, Kaye SJ, Martin RM, Davey Smith G, Cook DG, Bergstrom E, Black S, Wadsworth ME, Fall CH, Freudenheim JL, Nie J, Huxley RR, Kolacek S, Leeson CP, Pearce MS, Raitakari OT, Lisinen I, Viikari JS, Ravelli AC, Rudnicka AR, Strachan DP, Williams SM (2008) Does initial breastfeeding lead to lower blood cholesterol in adult life? A quantitative review of the evidence *Am J Clin Nutr* 88(2): 305-314

Owen CG, Whincup PH, Odoki K, Gilg JA, Cook DG (2002) Infant feeding and blood cholesterol: a study in adolescents and a systematic review. *Pediatrics* 110: 597-608

Owen CG, Whincup PH, Odoki K, Gilg JA, Cook DG (2003b) Birth weight and blood cholesterol level. a study in adolescents and systematic review. *Pediatrics* 111: 1081-1089

Owen CG, Whincup PH, Orfel L, Chou QA, Rudnicka AR, Wathern AK, Kaye SJ, Eriksson JG, Osmond C, Cook DG (2009b) Is body mass index before middle age related to coronary heart disease risk in later life? *Int J Obesity* 33(8): 866-877

Ozanne SE, Hales CN (2002) Early programming of glucose-insulin metabolism. *Trends Endocrinol Metab* 13: 368-373

Ozanne SE, Hales CN (2004) Lifespan: catch-up growth and obesity in male mice. *Nature* 427: 411-412

Paffenbarger RS, Wing AL (1969) Chronic disease in former college students. X. The effects of single and multiple characteristics on risk of fatal coronary heart disease. *Am J Epidemiol* 90: 527-535

Painter RC, De Rooij SR, Bossuyt PM, Osmond C, Barker DJ, Bleker OP, Roseboom TJ (2006) A possible link between prenatal exposure to famine and breast cancer: a preliminary study. *Am J Hum Biol* 18: 853-856

Painter RC, Roseboom TJ, van Montfrans GA, Bossuyt PM, Krediet RT, Osmond C, Barker DJ, Bleker OP (2005) Microalbuminuria in adults after prenatal exposure to the Dutch famine. *J Am Soc Nephrol* 16: 189-194

Paltiel O, Harlap S, Deutsch L, Knaanie A, Massalha S, Tiram E, Barchana M, Friedlander Y (2004) Birth weight and other risk factors for acute leukemia in the Jerusalem Perinatal Study cohort. *Cancer Epidemiol Biomarkers Prev* 13: 1057-1064

Paneth N, Susser M (1995) Early origin of coronary heart disease (the "Barker hypothesis"). *BMJ* 310: 411-412

Pardi G, Cetin I (2006) Human fetal growth and organ development: 50 years of discoveries. *Am J Obstet Gynecol*, 194(4): 1088-1099

Parsons TJ, Power C, Logan S, Summerbell CD (1999) Childhood predictors of adult obesity: a systematic review. *Int J Obes Relat Metab Disord* 23 Suppl 8: S1-S107

Pedersen J (1954) Weight and length at birth of infants of diabetic mothers. *Acta Endocrinol (Copenh)* 16: 330-342

Pedersen, J (1977) *The Pregnant Diabetic and Her Newborn – Problems and Management*. Copenhagen: Munksgaard.

Pelletier DL, Frongillo EA Jr, Habicht JP (1993) Epidemiologic evidence for a potentiating effect of malnutrition on child mortality. *Am J Public Health* 83: 1130-1133

Petridou E, Syrigou E, Toupadaki N, Zavitsanos X, Willet W, Trichopoulos D (1996) Determinants of age at menarche as early life predictors of breast cancer risk. *Int J Cancer* 68: 193-198

Petrie L, Duthie SJ, Rees WD, McConnell JM (2002) Serum concentrations of homocysteine are elevated during early pregnancy in rodent models of fetal programming. *Br J Nutr* 88: 471-477

Pettitt DJ, Forman MR, Hanson RL, Knowler WC, Bennett PH (1997) Breastfeeding and incidence of non-insulin-dependent diabetes mellitus in Pima Indians. *Lancet* 350: 166-168

Phipps K, Barker DJ, Hales CN, Fall CH, Osmond C, Clark PM (1993) Fetal growth and impaired glucose tolerance in men and women. *Diabetologia* 36: 225-228

Pietrobelli A, Faith MS, Allison DB, Gallagher D, Chiumello G, Heymsfield SB (1998) Body mass index as a measure of adiposity among children and adolescents: a validation study. *J Pediatr* 132: 204-210

Pisacane A, Graziano L, Mazzarella G, Scarpellino B, Zona G (1992) Breastfeeding and urinary tract infection. *J Pediatr* 120: 87-89

Platz EA, Giovannucci E, Rimm EB, Curhan GC, Spiegelman D, Colditz GA, Willett WC (1998) Retrospective analysis of birth weight and prostate cancer in the Health Professionals Follow-up Study. *Am J Epidemiol* 147: 1140-1144

Post WS, Goldschmidt-Clermont PJ, Wilhide CC, Heldman AW, Sussman MS, Ouyang P, Milliken EE, Issa JP (1999) Methylation of the estrogen receptor gene is associated with aging and atherosclerosis in the cardiovascular system. *Cardiovasc Res* 43: 985-991

Prader A, Tanner JM, von Harnack G (1963) Catch-up growth following illness or starvation. An example of developmental canalization in man. *J Pediatr* 62: 646-659

Prentice A (2003) Micronutrients and the bone mineral content of the mother, fetus and newborn. *J Nutr* 133: S1693-S1699

Prentice AM, Goldberg GR (1996) Maternal obesity increases congenital malformations. *Nutr Rev* 54: 146-50

Prentice AM, Goldberg GR (2000) Energy adaptations in human pregnancy: limits and long-term consequences. *Am J Clin Nutr* 71: S1226-S1232

Prentice A, Jarjou LM, Goldberg GR, Bennett J, Cole TJ, Schoenmakers I (2009) Maternal plasma 25-hydroxyvitamin D concentration and birthweight, growth and bone mineral accretion of Gambian infants. *Acta Paediatr* 988: 1360-1362

Prentice AM, Jebb SA (2003) Fast foods, energy density and obesity: a possible mechanistic link. *Obes Rev* 4: 187-194

Quigley MA, Kelly YJ, Sacker A (2007) Breastfeeding and hospitalization for diarrhoeal and respiratory infection in the United Kingdom Millennium Cohort Study. *Pediatrics* 119: e837-e842

Rao S, Yajnik CS, Kanade A, Fall CH, Margetts BM, Jackson AA, Shier R, Joshi S, Rege S, Lubree H, Desai B (2001) Intake of micronutrient-rich foods in rural Indian mothers is associated with size of their babies at birth: Pune Maternal Nutrition Study. *J Nutr* 131: 1217-1224

Rasmussen KM (2001) The "fetal origins" hypothesis: challenges and opportunities for maternal and child nutrition. *Annu Rev Nutr* 21: 73-95

Rasmussen SA, Chu SY, Kim SY, Schmid CH, Lau J (2008) Maternal obesity and risk of neural tube defects: a metaanalysis. *Am J Obstet Gynecol* 198: 611-619

Rasmussen KM, Yaktine AL (2009) *Weight Gain During Pregnancy: Reexamining the Guidelines*. Food and Nutrition Board and Board on Children, Youth and Families. Washington, DC: The National Academies Press.

Ravelli AC, van der Meulen JH, Michels RP, Osmond C, Barker DJ, Hales CN, Bleker OP (1998) Glucose tolerance in adults after prenatal exposure to famine. *Lancet* 351: 173-177

Ravelli AC, van der Meulen JH, Osmond C, Barker DJ, Bleker OP (2000) Infant feeding and adult glucose tolerance, lipid profile, blood pressure, and obesity. *Arch Dis Child* 82: 248-252

Ray JG, Wyatt PR, Vermuelen MJ, Meier C, Cole DE (2005) Greater maternal weight and the ongoing risk of neural tube defects after folic acid flour fortificaton. *Obstet Gynecol* 105: 261-265

Rees GA, Brooke Z, Doyle W, Costeloe K (2005a) The nutritional status of women in the first trimester of pregnancy attending an inner-city antenatal department in the UK. *J R Soc Health* 125: 232-238

Rees GA, Doyle W, Srivastava A, Brooke ZM, Crawford MA, Costeloe KL (2005b) The nutrient intakes of mothers of low birth weight babies – a comparison of ethnic groups in East London, UK. *Matern Child Nutr* 1: 91-99

Reik W, Constancia M, Fowden A, Anderson N, Dean W, Ferguson-Smith A, Tycko B, Sibley C (2003) Regulation of supply and demand for maternal nutrients in mammals by imprinted genes. *J Physiol* 547(1): 35-44

Reik W, Dean W, Walter J (2001) Epigenetic reprogramming in mammalian development. *Science* 293 (5532): 1089-1093

Reilly JJ, Armstrong J, Dorosty AR, Emmett PM, Ness A, Rogers I, Steer C, Sherriff A (2005) Early life risk factors for obesity in childhood: cohort study. *BMJ* 330: 1357

Relton CL, Pearce MS, Parker L (2005) The influence of erythrocyte folate and serum vitamin B12 status on birth weight. *Br J Nutr* 93: 593-599

Remacle C, Bieswal F, Reusens B (2004) Programming of obesity and cardiovascular disease. *Int J Obes Relat Metab Disord* 28 Suppl 3: S46-S53

Rich-Edwards JW, Kleinman K, Michels KB, Stampfer MJ, Manson JE, Rexrode KM, Hibert EN, Willett WC (2005) Longitudinal study of birth weight and adult body mass index in predicting risk of coronary heart disease and stroke in women. *BMJ* 330: 1115

Robinson S, Crozier SR, Borland SE, Hammond J, Barker DJP, Inskip HM (2004) Impact of educational attainment on the quality of young women's diets. *Eur J Clin Nutr* 58(8): 1174-1180

Robinson S, Crozier SR, Marriott L, Harvey N, Inskip HM, Godfrey K, Cooper C (2008) Impact of educational attainment on the quality of young women's diets. *Proc Nutr Soc* 67 (OCE8): E347

Robinson S, Godfrey K, Osmond C, Cox V, Barker D (1996) Evaluation of a food frequency questionnaire used to assess nutrient intakes in pregnant women. *Eur J Clin Nutr* 50: 302-308

Robinson S, Godfrey K, Denne J, Cox V (1998) The determinants of iron status in early pregnancy. *Br J Nutr* 79: 249-255

Robinson SM, Marriott LD, Crozier SR, Harvey NC, Gale CR, Inskip HM, Baird J, Law CM, Godfrey KM, Cooper C; Southampton Women's Survey Study Group (2009) Variations in infant feeding practice are associated with body composition in childhood: a prospective cohort study. *J Clin Endocrinol Metab* 94: 2799-2805

Robinson JS, Owens JA, de Barro T, Lok F (1994) *Maternal nutrition and fetal growth.* In: *Early fetal growth and development*, Ward RHT, Smith SK, Donnai D (eds). London: Royal College of Obstetricians and Gynaecologists.

Rogers I (2003) The influence of birth weight and intrauterine environment on adiposity and fat distribution in later life. *Int J Obes Relat Metab Disord* 27: 755 777

Rogers I, Emmett P, the ALSPAC Study Team (1998) Diet during pregnancy in a population of pregnant women in South West England. *Eur J Clin Nutr* 52: 246-250

Rogers I, Metcalfe C, Gunnell D, Emmett P, Dunger D, Holly J, and the Avon Longitudinal Study of Parents and Children Study Team (2006) Insulin-like growth factor-I and growth in height, leg length, and trunk length between ages 5 and 10 years. *J Clin Endocrinol Metab* 91: 2514-2519

Roseboom TJ, van der Meulen JH, Osmond C, Barker DJ, Ravelli AC, Bleker OP (2000a) Plasma lipid profiles in adults after prenatal exposure to the dutch famine. *Am J Clin Nutr* 72: 1101-1106

Roseboom TJ, van der Meulen JH, Osmond C, Barker DJ, Ravelli AC, Schroeder-Tanka JM, van Montfrans GA, Michels RP, Bleker OP (2000b) Coronary heart disease after prenatal exposure to the dutch famine, 1944-45. *Heart* 84: 595-598

Roseboom TJ, van der Meulen JH, Ravelli AC, Osmond C, Barker DJ, Bleker OP (2000c) Plasma fibrinogen and factor VII concentrations in adults after prenatal exposure to famine. *Br J Haematol* 111: 112-117

Roseboom TJ, van der Meulen JH, Ravelli AC, van Montfrans GA, Osmond C, Barker DJ, Bleker OP (1999) Blood pressure in adults after prenatal exposure to famine. *J Hypertens* 17. 325-330

Roseboom TJ, van der Meulen JH, van Montfrans GA, Ravelli AC, Osmond C, Barker DJ, Bleker OP (2001) Maternal nutrition during gestation and blood pressure in later life. *J Hypertens* 19: 29-34

Roseboom TJ, de Rooij S, Painter R (2006) The Dutch famine and its long-term consequences for adult health. *Early Human Dev* 82: 485-491

Ruston D, Hoare J, Henderson L, Gregory J, Bates CJ, Prentice A, Birch M, Swan G, Farron M (2004) *National Diet and Nutrition Survey: adults aged 19-64 years. Volume 4: Nutritional Status (anthropometry and blood analytes), blood pressure and physical activity.* London: The Stationery Office.

Sandhu MS, Luben R, Day NE, Khaw KT (2002) Self-reported birth weight and subsequent risk of colorectal cancer. *Cancer Epidemiol Biomarkers Prev* 11: 935-938

Savino F, Fissore MF, Grassino EC, Nanni GE, Oggero R, Silvestro L (2005) Ghrelin, leptin and IGF-I levels in breast-fed and formula-fed infants in the first years of life. *Acta Paediatr* 94: 531-537

Sayers A, Tobias JH (2009) Estimated maternal ultravioletB exposure levels in pregnancy influence skeletal development of the child. *J Clin Endocrinol Metab* 94: 765-771

Schack-Nielsen L, Michaelsen KF (2007) Advances in our understanding of the biology of human milk and its effects on the offspring. *J Nutr* 137: S503-S510

Schluchter MD (2003) Publication bias and heterogeneity in the relationship between systolic blood pressure, birth weight, and catch up growth – a meta analysis. *J Hyperten* 21: 273-279

Schmidt IM, Jørgensen MH, Michaelsen KF (1995) Height of conscripts in Europe: is postneonatal mortality a predictor? *Ann Hum Biol* 22: 57-67

Scholl TO, Chen X, Gaughan C, Smith WK (2002) Influence of maternal glucose level on ethnic differences in birth weight and pregnancy outcome. *Am J Epidemiol* 156: 498-506

Scholl TO, Chen X, Khoo CS, Lenders C (2004) The dietary glycemic index during pregnancy: influence on infant birth weight, fetal growth, and biomarkers of carbohydrate metabolism. *Am J Epidemiol* 159: 467-474

Scholl TO, Hediger ML, Khoo CS, Healey MF, Rawson NL (1991) Maternal weight gain, diet and infant birth weight: correlations during adolescent pregnancy. *J Clin Epidemiol* 44: 423-428

Scholl TO, Hediger ML, Schall JI, Khoo CS, Fischer RL (1994) Maternal growth during pregnancy and the competition for nutrients. *Am J Clin Nutr* 60: 183-188

Scholl TO, Sowers M, Chen X, Lenders C (2001) Maternal glucose concentration influences fetal growth, gestation, and pregnancy complications. *Am J Epidemiol* 154: 514-520

Scholl TO, Johnson WG (2000) Folic acid: influence on the outcome of pregnancy. *Am J Clin Nutr* 71: S1295-S1303

Schrezenmeir J, Jagla A (2000) Milk and diabetes. *J Am Coll Nutr* 19: S176-S190

Scientific Advisory Committee on Nutrition (2002) *A framework for the Evaluation of Evidence*. Accessed online at: http://www.sacn.gov.uk/pdfs/sacn_02_02a.pdf.

Scientific Advisory Committee on Nutrition (2004) *Advice on fish consumption: benefits & risks*. London: The Stationery Office.

Scientific Advisory Committee on Nutrition (2006) *Folate and disease prevention*. London: The Stationery Office.

Scientific Advisory Committee on Nutrition (2007a) *Application of WHO growth standards in the UK*. London: The Stationery Office.

Scientific Advisory Committee on Nutrition (2007b) *Update on Vitamin D*. London: The Stationery Office.

Scientific Advisory Committee on Nutrition (2008a) *Infant feeding survey 2005: A commentary on infant feeding practices in the UK*. London: The Stationery Office.

Scientific Advisory Committee on Nutrition (2008b) *Consideration of nutritional requirements in multiple pregnancies*. Accessed online at: http://www.sacn.gov.uk/pdfs/SACN%20Statement%20-%20Multiple%20Pregnancies%20FINAL%2018.06.08.pdf

Scientific Advisory Committee on Nutrition (2008c) *The nutritional health of the British population*. London: The Stationery Office.

Scientific Advisory Committee on Nutrition (2010) *Iron and Health*. London: The Stationery Office.

Scientific Advisory Committee on Nutrition (2009b) *Summary of Report to CMO on folic acid and colorectal cancer risk*. Accessed online at: http://www.sacn.gov.uk/reports_position_statements/reports/summary_of_report_to_cmo_on_folic_acid_and_colorectal_cancer_risk_-_october_2009.html

Sebire NJ, Jolly M, Harris JP, Wadsworth J, Joffe M, Beard RW, Regan L, Robinson S (2001) Maternal obesity and pregnancy outcome: a study of 287,213 pregnancies in London. *Int J Obes Relat Metab Disord* 25: 1175-1182

Seckl JR (1998) Physiologic programming of the fetus. *Clin Perinatol* 25: 939-62, vii

Seckl JR, Meaney MJ (2004) Glucocorticoid programming. *Ann N Y Acad Sci* 1032: 63-84

Shah A, Sands J, Kenny L (2005) Maternal obesity and the risk of still birth and neonatal death. *J Obstet Gynaecol* 26(1): S19

Shah PS, Shah V (2009) Influence of the maternal birth status on offspring: a systematic review and meta-analysis. *Acta Obstet Gynecol Scand.* 88(12): 1307-1318

Shehadeh N, Shamir R, Berant M, Etzioni A (2001) Insulin in human milk and the prevention of type 1 diabetes. *Pediatr Diabetes* 2: 175-177

Shenoy SD, Swift P, Cody D, Iqbal J (2005) Maternal vitamin D deficiency, refractory neonatal hypocalcaemia, and nutritional rickets. *Arch Dis Child* 90: 437-438

Sibley CP (2009) Understanding placental nutrient transfer – why bother? New biomarkers of fetal growth. *J Physiol* 587: 3431-3440

Sibley CP, Turner MA, Cetin I, Ayuk P, Boyd CA, D'Souza SW, Glazier JD, Greenwood SL, Jansson T, Powell T (2005) Placental phenotypes of intrauterine growth. *Pediatr Res* 58: 827-832

Simell O, Niinikoski H, Ronnemaa T, Lapinleimu H, Routi T, Lagstrom H, Salo P, Jokinen E, Viikari J (2000) Special Turku Coronary Risk Factor Intervention Project for Babies (STRIP). *Am J Clin Nutr* 72: S1316-S1331

Sinclair D (1989) *Human Growth After Birth, 5th Edition*. Oxford: Oxford University Press.

Singhal A, Cole TJ, Fewtrell M, Lucas A (2004) Breastmilk feeding and lipoprotein profile in adolescents born preterm: follow-up of a prospective randomised study. *Lancet* 363: 1571-1578

Singhal A, Cole TJ, Lucas A (2001) Early nutrition in preterm infants and later blood pressure: two cohorts after randomised trials. *Lancet* 357: 413-419

Singhal A, Fewtrell M, Cole TJ, Lucas A (2003) Low nutrient intake and early growth for later insulin resistance in adolescents born preterm. *Lancet* 361: 1089-1097

Singhal A, Lucas A (2004) Early origins of cardiovascular disease: is there a unifying hypothesis? *Lancet* 363: 1642-1645

Smith GD, Shipley MJ, Rose G (1990) Magnitude and causes of socioeconomic differentials in mortality: further evidence from the Whitehall Study. *J Epidemiol Community Health* 44: 265-270

Smuts CM, Huang M, Mundy D, Plasse T, Major S, Carlson SE (2003) A randomized trial of docosahexaenoic acid supplementation during the third trimester of pregnancy. *Obstet Gynecol* 101: 469-479

Snoeck A, Remacle C, Reusens B, Hoet JJ (1990) Effect of a low protein diet during pregnancy on the fetal rat endocrine pancreas. *Biol Neonate* 57: 107-118

Socha P, Janas R, Dobrzanska A, Koletzko B, Broekaert I, Brasseur D, Sengier A, Giovannini M, Agostoni C, Monasterolo RC, Mendezs G (2005) Insulin like growth factor regulation of body mass in breastfed and milk formula fed infants. Data from the E.U. Childhood Obesity Programme. *Adv Exp Med Biol* 569: 159-163

Sohlstrom A, Forsum E (1995) Changes in adipose tissue volume and distribution during reproduction in Swedish women as assessed by magnetic resonance imaging. *Am J Clin Nutr* 61: 287-295

Sorensen HT, Sabroe S, Rothman KJ, Gillman M, Fischer P, Sorensen TI (1997) Relation between weight and length at birth and body mass index in young adulthood: cohort study. *BMJ* 315: 1137

Specker B (2004) Vitamin D requirements during pregnancy. *Am J Clin Nutr* 80: S1740-S1747

Srinivasan SR, Bao W, Wattigney WA, Berenson GS (1996) Adolescent overweight is associated with adult overweight and related multiple cardiovascular risk factors: the Bogalusa Heart Study. *Metabolism* 45: 235-240

Stanner SA, Bulmer K, Andres C, Lantseva OE, Borodina V, Poteen VV, Yudkin JS (1997) Does malnutrition *in utero* determine diabetes and coronary heart disease in adulthood? Results from the Leningrad siege study, a cross sectional study. *BMJ* 315: 1342-1348

Stanner SA, Yudkin JS (2001) Fetal programming and the Leningrad Siege study. *Twin Res* 4: 287-292

Stein AD, Lumey LH (2000) The relationship between maternal and offspring birth weights after maternal prenatal famine exposure: the Dutch Famine Birth Cohort Study. *Hum Biol* 72: 641-654

Stein CE, Fall CH, Kumaran K, Osmond C, Cox V, Barker DJ (1996) Fetal growth and coronary heart disease in south India. *Lancet* 348: 1269-1273

Stein AD, Wang M, Ramirez-Zea M, Flores R, Grajeda R, Melgar P, Ramakrishnan U, Martorell R (2006) Exposure to a nutrition supplementation intervention in early childhood and risk factors for cardiovascular disease in adulthood: evidence from Guatemala. *Am J Epidemiol* 164: 1160-1170

Stein AD, Zybert PA, van de Bor M, Lumey LH (2004) Intrauterine famine exposure and body proportions at birth: the Dutch Hunger Winter. *Int J Epidemiol* 33: 831-836

Stephansson O, Dickman PW, Johansson A, Cnattingius S (2001) Maternal weight, pregnancy weight gain, and the risk of antepartum stillbirth. *Am J Obstet Gynecol* 184: 463-469

Stettler N (2007) Nature and strength of epidemiological evidence for origins of childhood and adulthood obesity in the first year of life. *Int J Obes* 31: 1035-1043

Stevens-Simon C, McAnarney ER, Roghmann KJ (1993) Adolescent gestational weight gain and birth weight. *Pediatrics* 92: 805-809

Stewart CP, Christian P, Schulze KJ, LeClerq SC, West KP, Khatry SK (2009) Antenatal micronutrient supplementation reduces metabolic syndrome in 6- to 8-year-old children in rural Nepal. *J Nutr* 139: 1575-81

Stratz CH (1904) *Der Korper des Kindes*. Fur Eltern, Arzta und Kunstler. Ferdinland Enke. Stuttgart: Germany

Stutz AM, Morrison CD, Argyropoulos G (2005) The agouti related protein and its role to homeostasis. *Peptides* 26: 1771-1781

Surani MA (2001) Reprogramming of genome function through epigenetic inheritance. *Nature* 414: 122-128

Susser M, Levin B (1999) Ordeals for the fetal programming hypothesis. The hypothesis largely survives one ordeal but not another. *BMJ* 318: 885-886

Symonds ME (2007) Integration of physiological and molecular mechanisms of the developmental origins of adult disease: new concepts and insights. *Proc Nutr Soc* 66: 442-450

Symonds ME, Budge H (2009) Nutritional models of the developmental origins of adult health and disease. *Proc Nutr Soc* 68: 173-178

Symonds ME, Budge H, Stephenson T (2000) Limitations of models used to examine the influence of nutrition during pregnancy and adult disease. *Arch Dis Child* 83: 215-219

Symonds ME, Sebert SP, Budge H (2009) The impact of diet during early life and its contribution to late disease: critical checkpoints in development and their long-term consequences for metabolic health. *Proc Nutr Soc* 68: 416-421

Szajewska H, Horvath A, Koletzko B (2006) Effect of *n*-3 long-chain polyunsaturated fatty acid supplementation of women with low-risk pregnancies on pregnancy outcomes and growth measures at birth: a meta-analysis of randomized controlled trials. *Am J Clin Nutr* 83: 1337-1344

Szyf M, Pakneshan P, Rabbani SA (2004) DNA methylation and breast cancer. *Biochem Pharmacol* 68: 1187-1197

Takai D, Jones PA (2002) Comprehensive analysis of CpG islands in human chromosome 21 and 22. *PNAS* 99(6): 3740-3745

Tamura T, Picciano MF (2006) Folate and human reproduction. *Am J Clin Nutr* 83: 993-1016

Tanner JM (1953) Growth of the human at the time of adolescence. *Lect Sci Basis Med.* 1: 308-363

Tanner JM (1978) *Fetus Into Man – Physical Growth from Conception to Maturity.* Cambridge, Massachusetts: Harvard University Press.

Tanner JM (1981) Catch-up growth in man. *Br Med Bull* 37: 233-238

Tanner JM (1990) *Foetus into man: physical growth from conception to maturity.* Ware: Castlemead Publications.

Tanner JM, Whitehouse RH, Marubini E, Resele LF (1976) The adolescent growth spurt of boys and girls of the Harpenden growth study. *Ann Hum Biol* 3: 109-126

Tanner JM, Whitehouse RH, Takaishi M (1966) Standards from birth to maturity for height, weight, height velocity, and weight velocity: British children, 1965. Part I. *Arch Dis Child* 41: 454-471

Tate AR, Dezateux C, Cole TJ, Millenium Cohort Study Child Health Group (2006) Is infant growth changing? *Int J of Obesity* 30: 1094-1096

Thame M, Trotman H, Osmond C, Fletcher H, Antoine M (2007) Body composition in pregnancies of adolescents and mature women and the relationship to birth anthropometry. *Eur J Clin Nutr* 61: 47-53

Thame M, Wilks R, Matadial L, Forrester TE (1999) A comparative study of pregnancy outcome in teenage girls and mature women. *West Indian Med J* 48: 69-72

Thame M, Wilks RJ, McFarlane-Anderson N, Bennett FI, Forrester TE (1997) Relationship between maternal nutritional status and infant's birth weight and body proportions at birth. *Eur J Clin Nutr* 51: 134-138

Thompson JR, FitzGerald P, Willoughby MLN, Armstrong BK (2001) Maternal folate supplementation in pregnancy and protection against acute lymphoblastic leukaemia in childhood: a case-control study. *Lancet* 358: 1935-1940

Thorsdottir I, Birgisdottir BE, Johannsdottir IM, Harris DP, Hill J, Steingrimsdottir L, Thorsson AV (2000) Different beta-casein fractions in Icelandic versus Scandinavian cow's milk may influence diabetogenicity of cow's milk in infancy and explain low incidence of insulin-dependent diabetes mellitus in Iceland. *Pediatrics* 106: 719-724

Tibblin G, Eriksson M, Cnattingius S, Ekbom A (1995) High birth weight as a predictor of prostate cancer risk. *Epidemiology* 6: 423-424

Tilling K, Davey Smith G, Chambless L, Rose K, Stevens J, Lawlor D, Szklo M (2004) The relation between birth weight and intima-media thickness in middle-aged adults. *Epidemiol* 15: 557-564

Tobias JH, Steer CD, Emmett PM, Tonkin RJ, Cooper C, Ness AR (2005) Bone mass in childhood is related to maternal diet in pregnancy. *Osteoporos Int* 16(12): 1731-1741

Tomat AL, Inserra F, Veiras L, Vallone MC, Balaszczuk AM, Costa MA, Arranz C (2008) Moderate zinc restriction during fetal and postnatal growth of rats: effects on adult arterial blood pressure and kidney. *Am J Physiol Regul Integr Comp Physiol* 295: R543-R549

Torrens C, Brawley L, Anthony FW, Dance CS, Dunn R, Jackson AA, Poston L, Hanson MA (2006) Folate supplementation during pregnancy improves offspring cardiovascular dysfunction induced by protein restriction. *Hypertension* 47: 982-987

Toschke AM, Martin RM, von Kries R, Wells J, Smith GD, Ness AR (2007) Infant feeding method and obesity: body mass index and dual-energy X-ray absorptiometry measurements at 9-10 y of age from the Avon Longitudinal Study of Parents and Children (ALSPAC). *Am J Clin Nutr* 85: 1578-1585

Tu YK, West R, Ellison GT, Gilthorpe MS (2005) Why Evidence for the Fetal Origins of Adult Disease Might Be a Statistical Artifact: The "Reversal Paradox" for the Relation between Birth Weight and Blood Pressure in Later Life. *Am J Epidemiol* 161: 27-32

Usha KTS, Hemmadi J, Bethel J, Evans J (2005) Outcome of pregnancy in women with an increased body mass index. *Br J Obstet Gynaecol* 112: 768-772

Vaidya A, Saville N, Shrestha BP, Costello AM, Manandhar DS, Osrin D (2008) Effects of a maternal multiple micronutrient supplement on children's weight and size at 2 years of age in Nepal; follow-up of a double blind randomised controlled trial. *Lancet* 371: 452-454

van Eijsden M, Hornstra G, van der Wal MF, Vrijkotte TG, Bonsel GJ (2008a) Maternal *n-3*, *n-6*, and *trans* fatty acid profile early in pregnancy and term birth weight: a prospective cohort study. *Am J Clin Nutr* 87(4): 887-895

van Eijsden M, Smits LJ, van der Wal MF, Bonsel GJ (2008b) Association between short interpregnancy intervals and term birth weight: the role of folate depletion. *Am J Clin Nutr* 88(1): 147-153

Veena SR, Kumaran K, Swarnagowri MN, Jayakumar MN, Leary SD, Stein CE, Cox VA, Fall CH (2004) Intergenerational effects on size at birth in South India. *Paed Perinatal Epidemiol* 18: 361-370

Vehaskari VM, Aviles DH, Manning J (2001) Prenatal programming of adult hypertension in the rat. *Kidney Int* 59: 238-245

Victora CG, Barros F, Lima RC, Horta BL, Wells J (2003) Anthropometry and body composition of 18 year old men according to duration of breast feeding: birth cohort study from Brazil. *BMJ* 327: 901

Victora CG, Barros FC (2001) Commentary: The catch-up dilemma – relevance of Leitch's 'low-high' pig to child growth in developing countries. *Int J Epidemiol* 30: 217-220

Viegas OA, Scott PH, Cole TJ, Mansfield HN, Wharton P, Wharton BA (1982) Dietary protein energy supplementation of pregnant Asian mothers at Sorrento, Birmingham. I: Unselective during second and third trimesters. *Br Med J (Clin Res Ed)* 285: 589-592

Virtanen SM, Laara E, Hypponen E, Reijonen H, Rasanen L, Aro A, Knip M, Ilonen J, Akerblom HK (2000) Cow's milk consumption, HLA-DQB1 genotype, and type 1 diabetes: a nested case-control study of siblings of children with diabetes. Childhood diabetes in Finland study group. *Diabetes* 49: 912-917

Visalli N, Sebastiani L, Adorisio E, Conte A, De Cicco AL, D'Elia R, Manfrini S, Pozzilli P (2003) Environmental risk factors for type 1 diabetes in Rome and province. *Arch Dis Child* 88: 695-698

von Versen-Hoeynck FM, Powers RW (2007) Maternal-fetal metabolism in normal pregnancy and preeclampsia. *Front Biosci* 1(12): 2457-2470

Waaler HT (1984) Height, weight and mortality. The Norwegian experience. *Acta Med Scand Suppl* 679: 1-56

Wadsworth M, Butterworth S, Marmot M, Ecob R, Hardy R (2005) Early growth and type 2 diabetes: evidence from the 1946 British birth cohort. *Diabetologia* 48: 2505-2510

Wadsworth ME, Hardy RJ, Paul AA, Marshall SF, Cole TJ (2002) Leg and trunk length at 43 years in relation to childhood health, diet and family circumstances; evidence from the 1946 national birth cohort. *Int J Epidemiol* 31: 383-390

Walton A, Hammond J (1938) The maternal effect on growth and conformation in Shire horse-Shetland pony crosses. *Proc Roy Soc (Biol)* 125: 311-318

Wannamethee SG, Shaper AG, Whincup PH, Walker M (1998) Adult height, stroke, and coronary heart disease. *Am J Epidemiol* 148: 1069-1076

Wannamethee SG, Whincup PH, Shaper G, Walker M (1996) Influence of fathers' social class on cardiovascular disease in middle-aged men. *Lancet* 348: 1259-1263

Waterland RA, Jirtle RL (2003) Transposable elements: targets for early nutritional effects on epigenetic gene regulation. *Mol Cell Biol* 23: 5293-5300

Watkins ML, Rasmussen SA, Honein MA, Botto LD, Moore CA (2003) Maternal obesity and risk for birth defects. *Paediatrics* 111: 1152-1158

Weaver IC (2009) Epigenetic effects of glucocorticoids. *Semin Fetal Neonatal Med.* 14: 143-150

Weiderpass E, Braaten T, Magnusson C, Kumle M, Vainio H, Lund E, Adami HO (2004) A Prospective Study of Body Size in Different Periods of Life and Risk of Premenopausal Breast Cancer. *Cancer Epidemiol Biomarkers Prev* 13: 1121-1127

Weintrob N, Karp M, Hod M (1996) Short- and long-range complications in offspring of diabetic mothers. *J Diabetes Complications* 10: 294-301

Weiss JL, Malone FD, Emig D, Ball RH, Nyberg DA, Comstock CH, Saade G, Eddleman K, Carter SM, Craigo SD, Carr SR, D'Alton ME (2004) Obesity, obstetric complications and cesarean delivery rate – a population-based screening study. *Am J Obstet Gynecol* 190: 1091-1097

Wells JC (2000) A Hattori chart analysis of body mass index in infants and children. *Int J Obes* 24: 325-329

Wells JC (2009) Historical cohort studies and the early origins of disease hypothesis: making sense of the evidence. *Proceedings of the Nutrition Society* 68: 179-188

Wells JC (2007) The thrifty phenotype as an adaptive maternal effect. *Biol Rev Camb Philos Soc* 82: 143-172

Wells JC, Chomtho S, Fewtrell MS (2007a) Programming of body composition by early growth and nutrition. *Proc Nutr Soc* 66: 423-434

Wells JC, Davies PS (1998) Estimation of the energy cost of physical activity in infancy *Arch Dis Child* 78(2): 131-136

Wells JC, Treleaven P, Cole TJ (2007b) BMI compared with 3-dimensional body shape: the UK National Sizing Survey. *Am J Clin Nutr* 85: 419-425

Wells JC, Victora CG (2005) Indices of whole-body and regional adiposity for evaluating the metabolic load of obesity. *Int J Obes* 29: 483-489

Whincup PH (1998) Fetal origins of cardiovascular risk: evidence from studies in children. *Proc Nutr Soc* 57: 123-127

Whincup, PH (2001) Age of menarche in contemporary British teenagers. *BMJ* 322: 1095-1096

Whincup PH, Kaye SJ, Owen CG (2008) Birth weight and risk of type 2 diabetes: a systematic review. *JAMA* 300(24): 2886-2897

Whitehead RG, Paul AA (1984) Growth charts and the assessment of infant feeding practices in the western world and in developing countries. *Early Hum Dev* 9: 187-207

Whorwood CB, Firth KM, Budge H, Symonds ME (2001) Maternal undernutrition during early to mid gestation programs tissue-specific alterations in the expression of the glucocorticoid receptor, 11beta-hydroxysteroid dehydrogenase isoforms, and type 1 angiotensin ii receptor in neonatal sheep. *Endocrinol* 142: 2854-2864

Widdowson EM (1968) Growth and composition of the fetus and newborn. In: *The Biology of Gestation*. NS Assali, ed. New York: Academic Press.

Widdowson EM, McCance RA (1975) A review: new thoughts on growth. *Pediatr Res* 9: 154-156

Wilcox AJ (2001) On the importance – and the unimportance – of birth weight. *Int J Epidemiol* 30: 1233-1241

Wilcox MA, Newton CS, Johnson IR (1995) Paternal influences on birthweight. *Acta Obstet Gynaecol Scandinavia* 74: 15-18

Wilcox AJ, Russell IT (1986) Birth weight and perinatal mortality: III. Toward a new method of analysis. *Int J Epidemiol* 15: 188-196

Wingard DL, Criqui MH, Edelstein SL, Tucker J, Tomlinson-Keasey C, Schwartz JE, Friedman HS (1994) Is breast-feeding in infancy associated with adult longevity? *Am J Public Health* 84: 1458-1462

Wolff GL, Kodell RL, Moore SR, Cooney CA (1998) Maternal epigenetics and methyl supplements affect agouti gene expression in Avy/a mice. *FASEB J* 12: 949-957

Wootton SA, Jackson AA (1995) *Influence of undernutrition in early life on growth, body composition and metabolic competence*. In: *Early environment and later outcomes*. Society for the Study of Human Biology, Symposium, Henry CJK (ed). Cambridge, Cambridge University Press.

World Bank (2006) *Repositioning Nutrition as Central to Development: A Strategy for Large-Scale Action*. Accessed online at: http://web.worldbank.org/WBSITE/EXTERNAL/TOPICS/EXTHEALTHNUTRITIONANDPOPULATION/EXTNUTRITION/0,,contentMDK:20787550~menuPK:282580~pagePK:64020865~piPK:149114~theSitePK:282575,00.html

World Cancer Research Fund/American Institute for Cancer Research (2007) *Food, Nutrition, Physical Activity, and the Prevention of Cancer: a Global Perspective.* Washington DC: AICR.

World Health Organization (2005) *The World Health Report: make every mother and child count.* Geneva, Switzerland: World Health Organization.

World Health Organization (2006) *WHO Promoting Optimal Fetal Development: Report of a Technical Consultation.* Geneva, Switzerland: World Health Organization.

Wright CM, Matthews JN, Waterston A, Aynsley-Green A (1994) What is a normal rate of weight gain in infancy? *Acta Paediatr* 83(4): 351-356

Wynn AHA, Crawford MA, Doyle W, Wynn SW (1991) Nutrition of women in anticipation of pregnancy. *Nutr Health* 7: 69-88

Yajnik CS (2002) The lifecycle effects of nutrition and body size on adult adiposity, diabetes and cardiovascular disease. *Obes Rev* 3: 217-224

Yajnik CS, Deshpande SS, Jackson AA, Refsum H, Rao S, Fisher DJ, Bhat DS, Naik SS, Coyaji KJ, Joglekar CV, Joshi N, Lubree HG, Deshpande VU, Rege SS, Fall CHD (2008) Vitamin B12 and folate concentrations during pregnancy and insulin resistance in the offspring: the Pune Maternal Nutrition Study. *Diabetologia* 51: 29-38

Yajnik CS, Fall CH, Coyaji KJ, Hirve SS, Rao S, Barker DJ, Joglekar C, Kellingray S (2003) Neonatal anthropometry: the thin-fat Indian baby. The Pune Maternal Nutrition Study. *Int J Obes Relat Metab Disord* 27: 173-180

Yajnik CS, Deshpande SS, Panchanadikar AV, Naik SS, Deshpande JA, Coyaji KJ, Fall C, Refsum H (2005) Higher maternal plasma homocysteine concentrations at 28 weeks gestation predicts smaller offspring size in rural India; a pilot study. *Asia Pacific J Clin Nutr* 14: 179-181

Ying AK, Hassanain HH, Roos CM, Smiraglia DJ, Issa JJ, Michler RE, Caligiuri M, Plass C, Goldschmidt-Clermont PJ (2000) Methylation of the estrogen receptor-alpha gene promoter is selectively increased in proliferating human aortic smooth muscle cells. *Cardiovasc Res* 46: 172-179

Yliharsila H, Kajantie E, Osmond C, Forsen T, Barker DJP, Eriksson JG (2007) Birth size, adult body composition and muscle strength in later life. *Int J Obes* 31: 1392-1399

Young TK, Martens PJ, Taback SP, Sellers EA, Dean HJ, Cheang M, Flett B (2002) Type 2 diabetes mellitus in children: prenatal and early infancy risk factors among native canadians. *Arch Pediatr Adolesc Med* 156: 651-655

Appendix 1 – Reviewing the evidence from epidemiological studies

1. Most of the data relating maternal, fetal and child exposures to CHD risk in humans is based on observational studies. Randomised controlled trials in this area, although providing support for the role of early exposures [Singhal *et al.*, 2001; Singhal *et al.*, 2003] have been limited in scope, duration and completeness of follow-up; serious ethical issues prevent the conduct of further early intervention trials [Barker, 1998].

2. The results of observational studies relating maternal, fetal and child exposures to CHD risk are therefore particularly important. A more systematic approach to interpretation of the observational study evidence on maternal, fetal and child influences on CHD risk, based on quantitative systematic reviews and meta-analysis of data from all observational studies (both published and unpublished) may help to overcome many of the difficulties in the interpretation of individual studies referred to above.

3. By identifying data from a large number of studies of different sizes, inconsistencies in study results due to small study size and statistical power can be resolved. The influence of adjustment (or lack of adjustment) for confounding factors and for current body size can be examined. In addition, the extent of publication bias (which usually results from the selective publication of small studies with extreme results) can be formally examined, and (if appropriate) the analyses limited to studies unlikely to have been affected by the results of publication bias (particularly large studies) so that the true strengths of association can be estimated.

4. Although the interpretation of systematic reviews of observational studies needs to be more cautious than that of randomized controlled trials [Egger *et al.*, 2001], the approach is potentially important in situations in which randomized controlled trial data are limited and a balanced view of the evidence is needed.

5. The use of quantitative systematic reviews offers several particular strengths. These strengths are outlined in the paragraphs below.

a) Opportunity to examine agreement/disagreement between studies

6. Differences between the estimates provided by different studies (heterogeneity) can be formally examined. Of particular importance is the opportunity to examine differences in the strength of associations by age of outcome — the concept of programming suggests that associations between maternal, fetal and child exposures and CHD risk might become more marked with increasing age [Law *et al.*, 1993]. An understanding of other reasons for differences in the strength of associations between studies may be extremely important. Particularly important

issues to examine are whether early life factor-CHD associations differ in strength between males and females, between populations in 'developing' and 'developed' countries, between populations of differing ethnic origin and between populations with differing prevalence of adult risk factors (e.g. prevalence of obesity or higher blood cholesterol concentrations in middle-age). Analyses conducted in relation to date of exposure could be particularly important when the nature of exposures have changed over time (e.g. changes in the composition of infant feeds) [Oppe, 1980; Oppe, 1974]; they could also be used to assess the contemporary relevance of specific maternal, fetal and child exposures [Whincup, 1998].

b) Opportunity to examine effects of study quality

7. The use of sensitivity analyses, restricting analyses to studies of high methodological quality and (where appropriate) the use of quality scores, allows the impact of study quality on the results to be formally examined.

c) High statistical power and precision

8. When pooled estimates can be derived from several different studies, these will normally provide considerably more precise estimates of the overall strength of relationships between maternal, fetal and child factors and CHD outcomes than can be obtained from any individual study. For example, in a recent meta-analysis of the association between birth weight and cholesterol, the 95% confidence intervals around the pooled regression estimate from all studies was only about half of that from the largest individual study [Owen et al., 2003b].

Appendix 2 – Maternal and child nutrition in the UK – National diet and nutrition data and smaller studies of pregnant women

1. SACN reviewed findings from the National Diet and Nutrition Surveys (NDNS) carried out between 1992 and 2001 [Scientific Advisory Committee on Nutrition, 2008c], and assessed the adequacy of dietary intakes by comparison with Dietary Reference Values (DRVs) set by the Committee on Medical Aspects of Food and Nutrition Policy (COMA) in 1991 [Department of Health, 1991]. The Low Income Diet and Nutrition Survey (LIDNS) also provides data on the dietary habits and biochemical status of the low income (materially deprived)[xlii] population in the UK [Nelson et al., 2007]. The Committee has focused on key findings from these surveys for young women of childbearing age and children aged 2-18 years. Evidence from small British studies of pregnant women are also described where available.

The diets of young children in the UK

Macronutrients

2. The NDNS showed mean energy intakes were below the EARs in all age groups (Table 1). Mean daily total energy intake in LIDNS was also similar to NDNS for boys and slightly higher for girls when comparing the 4-18 year age groups [Nelson et al., 2007].

3. The percentage of food energy from total carbohydrate, non-milk extrinsic sugars (NMES), protein, total fat, saturated fatty acids and trans fatty acids (as reported in NDNS) and comparison with the COMA Dietary Reference Values (DRVs) is shown in Table 2. Comparison of percentage of food energy from protein, carbohydrate and total fat between NDNS and LIDNS showed only small differences in the 4-18 year groups.

4. Mean NMES intakes exceeded the DRV (≤11% food energy) in all age groups in the NDNS with mean intakes up to 19% of food energy in the youngest age group; the main source of which was soft drinks. Mean intakes also exceeded the DRV in all age groups in LIDNS.

5. The NDNS showed mean non-starch polysaccharides (NSP) intakes in all age groups were below the DRV for adults (18g/day); mean intakes ranged from 6g/day for children <5 years to 12g/day for children 15-18 years (Table 4). In LIDNS, NSP intakes were also lower than the DRV in all age groups.

---

xlii   The Low Income Diet and Nutrition Survey (LIDNS) is based on a national sample of the most materially deprived households in the UK. "Low-income" used in the sections here on, refers to this population studied in the LIDNS.

Vitamins

6. The NDNS showed mean intakes of all vitamins except vitamin A were above RNIs[xliii] (Table 4). A tenth of children aged 1½-18 years had intakes below the LRNI [xliv], although there was little evidence of low vitamin A status based on plasma retinol levels except in the 1½-4½ year group (Table 8).

7. Mean vitamin D intakes from food for children under 5 years were 18% of the RNI. However, there was no evidence of low status in this group (Table 8). In older children, status indices for vitamin D indicate that 13% of 11-18 year-olds had low status (below the normal adult range). In LIDNS, mean daily intakes for vitamin D were 22% of the RNI for children aged 2-3 years (for whom an RNI is set).

8. In the NDNS, 16% of children under 4 years and 47% of girls aged 11-18 years had iron intakes below the LRNI (Table 10). A substantial proportion of both age groups were anaemic and/or had low iron stores (Table 11). LIDNS also showed that mean intakes of total iron fell below the RNI in girls aged 11-18 years and 40% of this age group had intakes below the LRNI.

9. In the NDNS a substantial number of children also had intakes for other minerals below the LRNI (Table 10). Similar findings were also observed in the LIDNS population.

Fruit & vegetables

10. The NDNS showed children aged 4-18 years consumed less than the recommendation for people aged over 5 years (≥400g/day) (Table 12). LIDNS also showed that mean fruit and vegetable consumption in children was well below the recommended levels.

Oily fish

11. In the NDNS, all age groups consumed well below the recommendation for oily fish consumption (≥1 portion per week) with mean consumption below 0.1 portion per week (Table 13). Only 3% of children in LIDNS reported eating oily fish and dishes containing oily fish.

The diet and nutritional status of young women of childbearing age

Macronutrients

12. Mean energy intakes and percentage of food energy from individual macronutrients as shown by the NDNS are given in Tables 1 and 2. Mean intakes of non-milk extrinsic sugars (NMES) and saturated fatty acids are above the DRV (both ≤11% of food energy). Findings were also similar in LIDNS for females (Table 3). Both the

---

xliii   Reference Nutrient Intake (RNI) is the average daily intake of a nutrient sufficient to meet the needs of almost all members (97.5%) of a healthy population. Values set may vary according to age, gender and physiological state (e.g. pregnancy or breastfeeding).

xliv   Lower Reference Nutrient Intake (LRNI) is the estimated average daily intake of a nutrient, which can be expected to meet the needs of only 2.5% of a healthy population. Values set may vary according to age, gender and physiological state (e.g. pregnancy or breastfeeding).

NDNS and LIDNS, and several British studies of pregnant women have found that average intakes of protein in pregnant women are above the RNI [xlv] [Haste et al., 1991; Wynn et al., 1991; Anderson et al., 1995; Robinson et al., 1996; Rogers et al., 1998].

13. Both the NDNS and LIDNS show that a high proportion of women in all age groups from 15-49 years were not consuming the minimum recommended amount of NSP (12g/day) (Table 5 and 6).

14. Both the NDNS and LIDNS show that most women in the UK consume very little fish (Table 13 and 14), where mean intake of oily fish in all age groups was below recommended levels [xlvi].

Fruit and vegetable consumption

15. The NDNS shows that a high proportion of young women consume less than the recommended "5 a day" [xlvii] (Table 12). This was also the case in LIDNS, and the mean number of portions consumed was lower in LIDNS, indicating a socio-economic gradient.

16. More recent trends data from the Health Survey for England 2009 also show that consumption of fruit and vegetables is below the recommended intake for women in the 16-44 years age group [Aresu et al., 2010], although these intakes are higher than that shown in the NDNS and LIDNS.

Micronutrients

17. The NDNS shows a high proportion of women aged 19-34 years and adolescent girls 15-18 years have low dietary intakes, and some evidence of low status for some micronutrients [Scientific Advisory Committee on Nutrition, 2008c]. This was also the case for several micronutrients in these age groups in LIDNS.

Folic acid

18. For pregnant women, the RNI for folate is 300μg/d (although during the first 12 weeks of pregnancy, this requirement is increased). Pregnant women have an increased requirement for folate and all women who could become pregnant are advised to take a 400μg/d folic acid supplement prior to conception and until the twelfth week of pregnancy, to reduce the risk of neural tube defects, such as spina bifida, in unborn babies [Scientific Advisory Committee on Nutrition, 2006].

---

xlv   There is a 6g/d increment in protein requirement for pregnant women through all stages of pregnancy [Department of Health, 1991].

xlvi   The population recommendation for fish consumption is for at least two portions of fish per week, of which one should be oily, subject to the restrictions on certain fish in pregnant and lactating women – marlin, swordfish, shark and, to a lesser extent, tuna – due to methylmercury contamination [Scientific Advisory Committee on Nutrition, 2004]. Fish, especially oily fish, contains long chain n-3 polyunsaturated fatty acids and a daily intake of 0.45g/d long chain n-3 polyunsaturated fatty acid is recommended [Scientific Advisory Committee on Nutrition, 2004].

xlvii   Dietary recommendations for adult consumption of fruit and vegetables advise eating at least five portions (400g) per day, and this is a universal recommendation for all adult population groups [Department of Health, 1991].

19.   Although the NDNS reported average daily folate intakes above the RNI for non-pregnant women in all age groups (Table 7), there was some evidence of marginal folate status in young women (Table 9). LIDNS also showed that relatively high proportions of the low-income population had low folate status. Several reports from British studies of pregnant women have also indicated that total folate intake is lower than the RNI for folate in pregnant women [Haste *et al.*, 1991; Wynn *et al.*, 1991; Anderson *et al.*, 1995; Robinson *et al.*, 1996; Mathews & Neil, 1998; Rogers *et al.*, 1998].

20.   A systematic review of dietary assessments of pregnant adolescents in industrialised countries found that folate intakes were low when compared to the US Dietary Reference Intake (DRI) (600µg per day), although the author acknowledged the poor quality of the majority of studies [Moran, 2007]. In addition, a prospective cohort of UK pregnant teenagers investigating associations with pregnancy outcome, found that folate intake was low among pregnant adolescents [Baker *et al.*, 2009].

21.   The 2005 Infant Feeding Survey (IFS) [Bolling *et al.*, 2007], based on retrospective postpartum interviews, found that almost eight in ten mothers reported they knew *why* increasing folic acid in the early stages of pregnancy was recommended; however, only half of these mentioned the reduced risk of spina bifida, and 13% mentioned neural tube defects when asked the reasons for increasing intake. The 2005 IFS also showed a high proportion of women were aware of the folic acid recommendation and took action to increase their folic acid intake during pregnancy, mostly by taking folic acid supplements. It is not clear from the survey, however, if they were taking supplements prior to conception as recommended.

22.   The Health Survey for England 2002 [Blake *et al.*, 2003] also provides information on the use of folic acid supplements prior to and during pregnancy. Of those mothers who reported planning their pregnancy, over half (55%) reported taking supplements or modifying their diet to increase folate intake before they became pregnant. Seventy-nine percent of mothers reported increasing their folate intake during pregnancy. The proportion of mothers taking action to address folate intake increased with age from 32% (16-24 years) to 60% (35 years and over). Only 43% of mothers in the most socioeconomically deprived areas were likely to increase their folate intake compared to 70% of mothers from the least socioeconomically deprived areas. LIDNS also showed that only 4% women in the 19-49 years age group took supplements containing folate [Nelson *et al.*, 2007].

23.   Research from the Southampton Women's Survey Study Group found that only a small proportion of women planning a pregnancy follow the recommendations for nutrition and lifestyle. This specifically showed that only 2.9% complied fully with the recommendation on folic acid intake in the three months before becoming pregnant. However, folic acid intakes from supplements were higher among the women who became pregnant within 3 months of the interview than those who did not. The percentages also increased in early pregnancy showing that considerably more women comply with the recommendation once they are pregnant [Inskip *et al.*, 2009].

Vitamin D

24. The vitamin D RNI for pregnant and lactating women is 10µg/d [Department of Health, 1991]. SACN recently emphasised the need for all pregnant and lactating women to consider taking a daily supplement of vitamin D, to ensure their own requirement for vitamin D is met, and to build adequate fetal stores for early infancy [Scientific Advisory Committee on Nutrition, 2007b].

25. National surveys have shown evidence for low vitamin D status in the general population (NDNS) and low-income groups (LIDNS), especially in younger women. Several British studies have reported that average vitamin D intakes were consistently lower than the RNI during pregnancy [Wynn et al., 1991; Anderson et al., 1995; Robinson et al., 1996; Mathews & Neil, 1998], although 25-hydroxyvitamin D (25(OH)D) is a more reliable measure of vitamin D status than intakes. A small study measuring serum 25(OH)D observed a high incidence of low vitamin D status in pregnant white women in the UK [Javaid et al., 2006]. Other studies in the UK have also reported low vitamin D status in Asian pregnant women [Datta et al., 2002; Shenoy et al., 2005], and it is well recognised that ethnic minority groups are particularly vulnerable to vitamin D deficiency [Scientific Advisory Committee on Nutrition, 2007b].

26. In addition, a prospective cohort of UK pregnant teenagers investigating associations with pregnancy outcome found that only a small fraction of pregnant teenagers consumed the recommended vitamin D intake [Baker et al., 2009].

27. There are no national data on the usage of vitamin D supplements in pregnant women, or of the uptake of Healthy Start vitamins, which contain vitamin D. A study of white women and their offspring (n=198) in Southampton [Javaid et al., 2006] reported that only 15% of mothers took a supplement containing vitamin D during pregnancy. A further prospective survey also highlighted that recommendations for vitamin D supplementation are ignored [Callaghan et al., 2006] and other studies have shown that there appears to be a lack of awareness of the recommendations to take vitamin D supplements in high risk groups [Allgrove, 2004; Shenoy et al., 2005]. However, information from the NHS Supply Chain and from invoices submitted to the Department of Health by individual PCTs, suggests that uptake of Healthy Start vitamins (containing vitamin D) is increasing [Department of Health, 2008].

Iron

28. There are no national data on the iron status of pregnant women, but national surveys of non-pregnant women of childbearing age show that average intakes are below the RNI for iron (Table 10). There is a high percentage of females aged 15-49 years with anaemia and poor iron status (Table 11). Several small British studies of pregnant women reported that mean iron intakes were below the RNI [Haste et al., 1991; Wynn et al., 1991; Anderson et al., 1995; Robinson et al., 1996; Rogers et al., 1998].

29. There is a lack of data on the prevalence of iron deficiency in pregnancy, but the prevalence of anaemia (low haemoglobin concentration) in UK pregnant women is low [Murphy et al., 1986; Godfrey et al., 1991; Robinson et al., 1998].

30. In the 2005 Infant Feeding Survey, 29% of women questioned postnatally reported taking an iron only supplement during pregnancy, while a further 17% took iron combined with vitamins [Bolling et al., 2007] and in the ALSPAC study of a cohort in Avon, 43% of women were consuming iron supplements at 32 weeks gestation [Rogers et al., 1998].

Other micronutrients

31. The NDNS shows that high proportions of women of child-bearing age, especially those aged 15-24 years, have intakes below the LNRI for vitamin A, riboflavin, iron, calcium, magnesium, potassium and iodine (Table 7 and 10). The NDNS also showed relatively high proportions had low biochemical status for riboflavin, vitamin B6 and to a lesser extent vitamin B_{12} (Table 9). Relatively high proportions of women in LIDNS had low biochemical status for vitamin C and folate, and to a lesser extent vitamin B_{12}.

32. The NDNS showed average intakes of salt (based on 24 hour urine collections) were higher than recommended in all women aged 19-49 years. Intake data for adolescent girls (not based on 24 hour urine collection) show that intakes are also above recommended in this age group[xlviii]. In LIDNS, salt intakes (again not based on 24 hour urine collection) were lower, but LIDNS excludes salt added at the table or in cooking, and these values are, therefore, an underestimate in most cases.

33. Several small studies have reported low micronutrient intakes in pregnant women in the UK, particularly those from more socially deprived areas [Rees et al., 2005a; Rees et al., 2005b; Mouratidou et al., 2006]. Some studies in pregnant women have shown intakes below the RNI for magnesium, potassium and vitamin B6 [Haste et al., 1991; Wynn et al., 1991; Anderson et al., 1995; Rogers et al., 1998]. Other studies have shown that recommended intakes in pregnant women are met for magnesium, vitamin B6, riboflavin, zinc and calcium [Haste et al., 1991; Wynn et al., 1991; Anderson et al., 1995; Robinson et al., 1996; Mathews & Neil, 1998; Rogers et al., 1998].

xlviii   Urinary sodium excretion provides a more reliable marker of sodium intake, but urinary data are not currently available for adolescent girls.

Appendix 2 Tables

The following tables are taken from the 2008 SACN report *The Nutritional Wellbeing of the British Population* [Scientific Advisory Committee on Nutrition, 2008c] which summarises data from the National Diet and Nutrition Surveys [Gregory *et al.*, 1995; Finch *et al.*, 1998; Gregory *et al.*, 2000; Henderson *et al.*, 2002; Henderson *et al.*, 2003a; Henderson *et al.*, 2003b; Ruston *et al.*, 2004] and the Low Income Diet and Nutrition Survey (LIDNS) [Nelson *et al.*, 2007].

Table 1   Average daily total energy intake (MJ) as a percentage of the estimated average requirement (EAR) by sex and age of respondent (NDNS)

Gender and age of respondent	Mean energy intake (MJ)	Intake as % EAR**	Number of subjects
Males and females aged 1½-2½ years***	4.39	90%	538
Males and females aged 2½-3½ years***	4.88	84%	578
Males aged (years)			
3½-4½***	5.36	82%	250
4 – 6	6.39	89%	184
7 – 10	7.47	91%	256
11- 14	8.28	89%	237
15 – 18	9.60	83%	179
19 – 24	9.44	89%	61
25 – 34	9.82	93%	160
35 – 49	9.93	94%	303
50 – 64	9.55	92%	242
65+ Free-living	8.02	85%	632
65+ Living in an institution	8.14	91%	204
Females aged (years)			
3.5-4.5***	4.98	82%	243
4-6	5.87	91%	171
7-10	6.72	92%	226
11-14	7.03	89%	238
15-18	6.82	77%	210
19-24	7.00	86%	78
25-34	6.61	82%	211
35-49	6.96	86%	379
50-64	6.91	87%	290
65+ Free-living	5.98	76%	643
65+ Living in an institution	6.94	90%	208

** Standard EAR values used for each age/sex group as published in the UK Dietary Reference Values.   EAR values for each age/sex group were derived from BMR calculated from the modified Schofield equations using mean body weight values for each age/sex group. PAL for adults taken as 1.4. The Estimated Average Requirements (EARs) for energy used are:

Men:
4-6 years: 7.16 MJ/day
7-10 years: 8.24 MJ/day
11-14 years 9.27 MJ/day
15-18 years 11.51 MJ/day
19 to 50 years: 10.60 MJ/d
51 to 59 years: 10.60 MJ/d
60 to 64 years: 9.93MJ/d

Women:
6.46 MJ/day
7.28 MJ/day
7.92 MJ/day
8.83 MJ/day
19 to 50 years: 8.10MJ/d
51 to 59 years: 8.00MJ/d
60 to 64 years: 7.99MJ/d

Energy intake as a percentage of EAR was calculated for each respondent using the EAR appropriate for sex and age.

*** Energy intakes per kilogram body weight were compared with EAR per kg body weight to calculate intake as % of EAR.

Table 2 Percentage of food energy from total carbohydrate, non-milk extrinsic sugars (NMES), protein, total fat, saturated fatty acids and trans fatty acids and comparison with COMA Dietary Reference Values (DRVs) (NDNS)

Gender and age	Percentage food energy from:						No of subjects (unweighted)
	Total carbohydrate	NMES	Protein	Total fat	Saturated fatty acids	Trans fatty acids	
Males aged (years)							
1.5-4.5	51.4	18.8	12.8	35.7	16.2	1.7	848
4-6	51.6	16.2	12.9	35.5	14.8	1.3	184
7-10	52.4	17.5	12.4	35.2	14.3	1.4	256
11-14	51.7	16.9	13.1	35.2	13.8	1.3	237
15-18	50.5	15.8	13.9	35.9	13.9	1.4	179
19-24	49.0	17.4	14.9	36.0	13.5	1.2	61
25-34	47.7	13.9	16.5	35.8	13.2	1.2	160
35-49	47.5	13.1	16.7	35.9	13.5	1.2	303
50-64	47.4	12.2	17.0	35.6	13.4	1.2	242
65+ Free-living	48.2	13.2	16.1	35.7	14.6	1.5	632
65+ Living in an institution	50.8	17.9	14.1	35.1	15.2	1.7	204
Females aged (years)							
1.5-4.5	50.8	18.6	13.1	36.1	16.2	1.7	827
4-6	51.4	17.6	12.7	35.9	15.3	1.3	171
7-10	51.3	16.7	12.8	35.9	14.5	1.4	226
11-14	51.2	16.2	12.7	36.1	14.0	1.3	238
15-18	50.6	15.3	13.9	35.9	13.8	1.3	210
19-24	49.1	14.2	15.4	35.5	12.9	1.1	78
25-34	48.7	11.8	15.9	35.4	13.2	1.1	211
35-49	48.6	11.8	16.7	34.7	13.2	1.2	379
50-64	48.1	11.0	17.4	34.5	13.3	1.2	290
65+ Free-living	47.5	11.5	16.5	36.1	15.3	1.6	643
65+ Living in an institution	51.3	18.5	14.0	34.8	15.4	1.8	208

Dietary reference values (DRVs) are:
Total carbohydrate should make up more than 50% of food energy intake
NMES should make up less than 11% of food energy intake
Total fat should make up less than 35% of food energy intake
Saturated fats should make up less than 11% of food energy intake
Trans fatty acids should make up less than 2% of food energy intake

Table 3 Percentage of food energy from total carbohydrate (CHO), non-milk extrinsic sugars (NMES), total fat, saturated fatty acids (SFA) and trans fatty acids (TFA) in females aged 11-49 years in LIDNS

Age (years)	Percentage food energy					No of subjects (unweighted)
	Total CHO	NMES	Total fat	SFA	TFA	
11-18	50.4	16.3	36.3	13.5	1.2	215
19-34	50.1	15.6	34.8	13.0	1.2	483
35-49	48.1	12.6	35.5	13.6	1.2	494

Table 4   Mean non-starch polysaccharides intake (grams per day) (NDNS)

Gender and age	Mean intake (g)	Number of subjects (unweighted)
Males aged (years)		
1.5-4.5	6.3	848
4 – 6	9.1	184
7 – 10	10.3	256
11 – 14	11.6	237
15 –18	13.3	179
19 – 24	12.3	61
25 – 34	14.6	160
35 – 49	15.7	303
50 – 64	16.4	242
65+ *Free-living*	13.5	632
65+ *Living in an institution*	11.0	204
Females aged (years)		
1.5-4.5	5.9	827
4 – 6	8.0	171
7 – 10	9.8	226
11 – 14	10.2	238
15 –18	10.6	210
19 – 24	10.6	78
25 – 34	11.6	211
35 – 49	12.8	379
50 – 64	14.0	290
65+ Free-living	11.0	643
65+ Living in an institution	9.5	208

Table 5   The percentage with NSP intakes below 12g/day in females aged 19-49 years in NDNS

Age (years)	<12g NSP/day	No of subjects (unweighted)
19-24	67	78
25-34	57	211
35-49	47	379

Table 6   The percentage with NSP intakes below 12g/day in females aged 11-49 years in LIDNS

Age (years)	% intakes below 12g/day	No of subjects (unweighted)
11-18	61	215
19-34	72	483
35-49	72	494

Table 7　Mean intakes of vitamins from food as a percentage of Reference Nutrient Intake (RNI) and percentage below the Lower Reference Nutrient Intake (LRNI), by age and sex (NDNS)

| Vitamin | Males and females Age (years) | | Males aged (years) | | | | | | | |
| | 1½-4 | | 4-6 | | 7-10 | | 11-14 | | 15-18 | |
	Mean intake as % RNI	% below LRNI	Mean intake as % RNI	% below LRNI	Mean intake as % RNI	% below LRNI	Mean intake as % RNI	% below LRNI	Mean intake as % RNI	% below LRNI
Vitamin A (retinol equivalents) (µg)	128	8	114	8	101	9	93	13	88	12
Thiamin (mg)	154	0	181	-	202	-	189	0	173	-
Riboflavin (mg)	197	0	194	-	162	1	144	6	148	6
Niacin equivalents (mg)	197	-	207	-	216	0	200	0	203	-
Vitamin B₆ (mg)	170	1	189	-	194	-	182	1	180	0
Vitamin B₁₂ (µg)	560	-	499	-	395	-	372	0	330	-
Folate (µg)	184	0	151	-	141	-	123	1	152	-
Vitamin C (mg)	160	1	223	-	243	-	218	1	208	-
Vitamin D (µg)†	18	N/A	N/A	N/A	N/A	N/A	N/A	N/A	N/A	N/A
Number of subjects (unweighted)	1457		184		256		237		179	

| Vitamin | Females aged (years) | | | | | | | |
| | 4-6 | | 7-10 | | 11-14 | | 15-18 | |
	Mean intake as % RNI	% below LRNI	Mean intake as % RNI	% below LRNI	Mean intake as % RNI	% below LRNI	Mean intake as % RNI	% below LRNI
Vitamin A (retinol equivalents) (µg)	112	6	96	10	78	20	91	12
Thiamin (mg)	163	-	182	-	200	1	172	2
Riboflavin (mg)	175	-	137	1	120	22	118	21
Niacin equivalents (mg)	186	-	195	-	205	-	180	1
Vitamin B₆ (mg)	169	-	174	1	190	1	150	5
Vitamin B₁₂ (µg)	446	-	347	-	270	1	225	2
Folate (µg)	169	-	126	2	102	3	105	4
Vitamin C (mg)	217	0	245	-	202	1	185	0
Vitamin D (µg)†	N/A	N/A	N/A	N/A	N/A	N/A	N/A	N/A
Number of subjects (unweighted)	171		226		238		210	

† Vitamin D is also obtained from the action of sunlight on the skin. There are no DRVs specified for vitamin D intake for children aged 4 years and over.

Table 7 (continued)   Mean intakes of vitamins from food as a percentage of Reference Nutrient Intake (RNI) and percentage below the Lower Reference Nutrient Intake (LRNI), by age and sex (NDNS)

Vitamin	Males aged (years)							
	19-24		25-34		35-49		50-64	
	Mean intake as % RNI	% below LRNI	Mean intake as % RNI	% below LRNI	Mean intake as % RNI	% below LRNI	Mean intake as % RNI	% below LRNI
Vitamin A (retinol equivalents) (µg)	80	16	103	7	141	5	164	4
Thiamin (mg)	160	2	232	0	204	0	230	1
Riboflavin (mg)	129	8	163	1	168	2	169	3
Niacin equivalents (mg)	232	–	272	–	270	0	279	0
Vitamin B$_6$ (mg)	189	–	211	0	206	2	201	1
Vitamin B$_{12}$ (µg)	296	1	395	–	465	0	485	0
Folate (µg)	151	2	173	–	171	0	181	–
Vitamin C (mg)	162	–	185	0	221	–	236	–
Vitamin D (µg)†	N/A	N/A	N/A	N/A	N/A	N/A	N/A	N/A
Number of subjects (unweighted)	61		160		303		242	

Vitamin	Females aged (years)							
	19-24		25-34		35-49		50-64	
	Mean intake as % RNI	% below LRNI	Mean intake as % RNI	% below LRNI	Mean intake as % RNI	% below LRNI	Mean intake as % RNI	% below LRNI
Vitamin A (retinol equivalents) (µg)	78	19	98	11	112	8	136	5
Thiamin (mg)	181	–	194	2	190	1	200	1
Riboflavin (mg)	126	15	131	10	151	5	159	6
Niacin equivalents (mg)	246	2	240	–	263	1	270	0
Vitamin B$_6$ (mg)	165	5	158	1	170	2	177	2
Vitamin B$_{12}$ (µg)	266	1	264	1	325	1	378	0
Folate (µg)	114	3	117	2	128	2	134	2
Vitamin C (mg)	170	1	181	–	200	0	236	0
Vitamin D (µg)†	N/A	N/A	N/A	N/A	N/A	N/A	N/A	N/A
Number of subjects (unweighted)	78		211		379		290	

(LRNI), by age and sex (NDNS)

Males aged (years)

Vitamin	65-74 Free-living		75-84 Free-living		85+ Free-living		65-84 Institution		85+ Institution	
	Mean intake as % RNI	% below LRNI	Mean intake as % RNI	% below LRNI	Mean intake as % RNI	% below LRNI	Mean intake as % RNI	% below LRNI	Mean intake as % RNI	% below LRNI
Vitamin A (retinol equivalents) (μg)	173	4	160	6	149	2	147	1	157	–
Thiamin (mg)	170	–	179	1	174	1	N/A	1	168	1
Riboflavin (mg)	137	4	130	5	126	5	133	3	146	2
Niacin equivalents (mg)	208	–	215	1	199	0	N/A	–	194	0
Vitamin B$_6$ (mg)	169	2	167	1	150	3	N/A	1-2	150	1
Vitamin B$_{12}$ (μg)	427	–	367	1	320	–	327	–	333	–
Folate (μg)	141	0	125	1	117	4	117	4	118	5
Vitamin C (mg)	179	1	148	1	127	2	123	–	127	2
Vitamin D (μg)†	43	N/A	38	N/A	32	N/A	36	N/A	41	N/A
Number of subjects (unweighted)	271		265		96		128		76	

Females aged (years)

Vitamin	65-74 Free-living		75-84 Free-living		85+ Free-living		65-84 Institution		85+ Institution	
	Mean intake as % RNI	% below LRNI	Mean intake as % RNI	% below LRNI	Mean intake as % RNI	% below LRNI	Mean intake as % RNI	% below LRNI	Mean intake as % RNI	% below LRNI
Vitamin A (retinol equivalents) (μg)	161	4	165	5	152	4	156	1	164	–
Thiamin (mg)	153	–	166	–	157	1	N/A	–	153	0
Riboflavin (mg)	133	10	128	9	117	15	155	–	141	6
Niacin equivalents (mg)	214	–	200	–	183	1	207	–	184	0
Vitamin B$_6$ (mg)	170	2	150	2	140	6	170	–	150	0
Vitamin B$_{12}$ (μg)	307	1	300	1	233	4	300	–	307	–
Folate (μg)	108	4	101	7	92	11	105	2	94	8
Vitamin C (mg)	168	1	136	1	122	4	129	–	111	0
Vitamin D (μg)†	30	N/A	30	N/A	23	N/A	33	N/A	33	N/A
Number of subjects (unweighted)	256		217		170		91		117	

† Vitamin D is also obtained from the action of sunlight on the skin.

Table 8   Percentage of respondents with low status for fat-soluble vitamins (NDNS)

	Plasma retinol		Plasma 25-hydroxy-vitamin D	Tocopherol: cholesterol ratio	Number of subjects (unweighted)
	severely deficient (<0.35 μmol/l) %	marginal status (0.35-0.7 μmol/l) %	below lower limit of normal range (<25 nmol/l) %	below lower limit of normal range (<2.25) %	
Males aged (years)					
1.5-4.5	2*	11**	–	n/a	377-411
4-6	–	2	3	–	55-73
7-10	–	2	4	–	135-167
11-14	–	–	11	–	163-177
15-18	–	–	16	–	143-153
19-24	–	–	24	1	45
25-34	–	–	16	1	107-115
35-49	–	–	12	1	213-243
50-64	–	1	9	1	168-189
65+ *Free-living*	–	–	6	n/d	436-476
65+ *Living in an institution*	–	3	38	n/d	131-138
Females aged (years)					
1.5-4.5	2*	10**	1	n/a	360-405
4-6	–	3	2	–	49-76
7-10	–	2	7	–	108-133
11-14	–	–	11	–	145-164
15-18	–	0	10	–	155-162
19-24	–	–	28	–	44-47
25-34	–	–	13	2	146-154
35-49	–	–	15	1	278-296
50-64	–	–	11	3	191-206
65+ *Free-living*	–	0	10	n/d	416-451
65+ *Living in an institution*	–	–	37	n/d	113-120

* <0.5 μmol/l
** 0.5-0.75 μmol/l

Table 9 Percentage of respondents with low status for water soluble vitamins (NDNS)

	Plasma vitamin C	Red cell folate		Serum folate	Serum vitamin B$_{12}$	Thiamin (ETKAC)	Riboflavin (EGRAC)	Vitamin B$_6$ (EAATAC)	Number of subjects (unweighted)
	Biochemical depletion (<11μmol/l) %	severely deficient (<230nmol/l) %	marginal status (230-350 μmol/l) %	Deficient (<6.3 nmol/l) %	Lower limit of normal range (<118 pmol/l) %	Biochemical deficiency (>1.25) %	Marginal /deficient status (>1.3) %	biochemical deficiency (>2.0) %	
Males aged (years)									
1.5-4.5	3**	n/d	n/d	n/d	n/d	n/a	19	n/a	380-421
4-6	5	-	3	-	-	1	59	7	69-86
7-10	2	1	3	-	-	-	78	8	165-185
11-14	1	1	7	-	-	0	80	11	172-181
15-18	3	-	12	1	1	-	80	15	152-161
19-24	7	-	13	-	-	-	82	4	45
25-34	5	1	3	1	-	3	70	10	119
35-49	4	1	4	1	2	2	67	13	245
50-64	5	-	2	1	3	5	54	11	191
65+ Free-living	14	8	20†	16***	8	8	41	n/a	454-480
65+ Living in an institution	44	13	29†	40***	7	11	41	n/a	132-142
Females aged (years)									
1.5-4.5	2**	n/d	n/d	n/d	n/d	n/a	27	n/a	364-407
4-6	2	-	1	-	-	1	75	6	76-82
7-10	3	1	8	-	-	2	85	11	125-138
11-14	1	-	11	1	-	2	90	14	161-169
15-18	4	1	13	1	8	3	95	8	156-169
19-24	4	-	8	-	5	-	77	12	53
25-34	3	-	4	-	5	1	78	8	157
35-49	4	-	5	0	4	2	69	12	298
50-64	3	0	6	-	3	1	50	13	210
65+ Free-living	13	8	22†	14***	5	9	42	n/a	439-459
65+ Living in an institution	38	18	15†	38***	10	15	32	n/a	116-122

** Less than 10μmol/l;
*** Less than 7nmol/l;
†230-345μmol/l

Table 10 Mean intakes of minerals from food sources as a percentage of Reference Nutrient Intake (RNI) and percentage with intakes below the Lower Reference Nutrient Intake (LRNI), by age and sex (NDNS)

Mineral	Males and females aged (years)		Males aged (years)									
	1½-4		4-6		7-10		11-14		15-18			
	Mean intake as % RNI	% below LRNI	Mean intake as % RNI	% below LRNI	Mean intake as % RNI	% below LRNI	Mean intake as % RNI	% below LRNI	Mean intake as % RNI	% below LRNI		
Total iron (mg)	77	16	134	-	111	1	95	3	111	2		
Calcium (mg)	183	1	157	3	135	2	80	12	88	9		
Magnesium (mg)	159	0	143	3	97	2	78	28	85	18		
Potassium (mg)	187	0	177	-	107	-	77	10	81	15		
Zinc (mg)	87	14	85	12	88	5	79	14	92	9		
Iodine (µg)	170	3	156	2	140	1	124	3	139	1		
Copper (mg)**	119	N/A	117	N/A	116	N/A	112	N/A	106	N/A		
Number of subjects (unweighted)	1457		184		256		237		179			

Mineral	Females aged (years)							
	4-6		7-10		11-14		15-18	
	Mean intake as % RNI	% below LRNI	Mean intake as % RNI	% below LRNI	Mean intake as % RNI	% below LRNI	Mean intake as % RNI	% below LRNI
Total iron (mg)	119	1	96	3	60	45	58	50
Calcium (mg)	146	2	119	5	80	24	82	19
Magnesium (mg)	129	1	89	5	65	51	64	53
Potassium (mg)	161	-	101	1	68	19	62	38
Zinc (mg)	75	26	81	10	66	37	87	10
Iodine (µg)	143	2	119	3	92	13	96	10
Copper (mg)**	106	N/A	105	N/A	98	N/A	80	N/A
Number of subjects (unweighted)	171		226		238		210	

** no LRNI set for copper

Table 10 (continued): Mean intakes of minerals from food sources as a percentage of Reference Nutrient Intake (RNI) and percentage with intakes below the Lower Reference Nutrient Intake (LRNI), by age and sex (NDNS)

Mineral	Males aged (years)							
	19-24		25-34		35-49		50-64	
	Mean intake as % RNI	% below LRNI	Mean intake as % RNI	% below LRNI	Mean intake as % RNI	% below LRNI	Mean intake as % RNI	% below LRNI
Total iron (mg)	131	3	150	0	157	1	156	1
Calcium (mg)	123	5	145	2	149	2	147	2
Magnesium (mg)	86	17	103	9	106	7	106	9
Potassium (mg)	81	18	94	3	99	5	101	5
Zinc (mg)	95	7	108	2	111	4	109	3
Iodine (µg)	119	2	154	1	158	2	164	1
Copper (mg)**	95	N/A	114	N/A	128	N/A	126	N/A
Number of subjects (unweighted)	61		160		303		242	

Mineral	Females aged (years)							
	19-24		25-34		35-49		50-64	
	Mean intake as % RNI	% below LRNI	Mean intake as % RNI	% below LRNI	Mean intake as % RNI	% below LRNI	Mean intake as % RNI	% below LRNI
Total iron (mg)	60	42	62	41	69	27	122	4
Calcium (mg)	99	8	104	6	114	6	118	3
Magnesium (mg)	76	22	77	20	87	10	91	7
Potassium (mg)	67	30	68	30	78	16	82	10
Zinc (mg)	98	5	96	5	108	4	112	3
Iodine (µg)	93	12	103	5	116	4	127	1
Copper (mg)**	76	N/A	83	N/A	88	N/A	89	N/A
Number of subjects (unweighted)	78		211		379		290	

** no LRNI set for copper

187

Table 10 (continued) Mean intakes of minerals from food sources as a percentage of Reference Nutrient Intake (RNI) and percentage with intakes below the Lower Reference Nutrient Intake (LRNI), by age and sex (NDNS)

Males aged (years)

Mineral	65-74 Free-living		75-84 Free-living		85+ Free-living		65-84 Institution		85+ Institution	
	Mean intake as % RNI	% below LRNI	Mean intake as % RNI	% below LRNI	Mean intake as % RNI	% below LRNI	Mean intake as % RNI	% below LRNI	Mean intake as % RNI	% below LRNI
Total iron (mg)	128	–	124	2	120	4	110	4	110	5
Calcium (mg)	122	4	116	5	109	2	134	–	140	1
Magnesium (mg)	88	16	80	29	72	36	71	37	72	42
Potassium (mg)	81	14	72	23	66	34	70	27	69	28
Zinc (mg)	95	6	88	12	85	15	88	14	87	12
Iodine (µg)	137	1	129	2	119	4	139	1	137	2
Copper (mg)**	98	N/A	87	N/A	73	N/A	80	N/A	77	N/A
Number of subjects (unweighted)	271		265		96		128		76	

Females aged (years)

Mineral	65-74 Free-living		75-84 Free-living		85+ Free-living		65-84 Institution		85+ Institution	
	Mean intake as % RNI	% below LRNI	Mean intake as % RNI	% below LRNI	Mean intake as % RNI	% below LRNI	Mean intake as % RNI	% below LRNI	Mean intake as % RNI	% below LRNI
Total iron (mg)	103	4	97	6	89	10	99	4	90	8
Calcium (mg)	101	8	97	10	92	15	129	1	118	1
Magnesium (mg)	77	19	69	27	66	34	74	16	66	27
Potassium (mg)	66	30	60	47	56	57	65	33	58	50
Zinc (mg)	100	3	96	7	91	10	107	1	96	6
Iodine (µg)	109	6	103	4	102	7	129	1	121	1
Copper (mg)**	76	N/A	69	N/A	66	N/A	72	N/A	68	N/A
Number of subjects (unweighted)	256		217		170		91		117	

** no LRNI set for copper

Table 11 Percentage of respondents below thresholds for iron status (NDNS)

Gender and age	Haemoglobin concentration	% Iron saturation	Serum ferritin	Number of subjects (unweighted)
	lower threshold for anaemia %	lower threshold for anaemia %	low iron stores %	
Male aged (years)				
1.5-4.5	7	n/a	24	475/-/467
4-6	3	23	18†	86/60/69
7-10	47	18	14	185/150/147
11-14	30	19	17	181/166/153
15-18	1	12	5	164/149/131
19-24	-	6	4	45/45/45
25-34	2	13	0	119/115/119
35-49	4	3	6	245/243/245
50-64	3	6	5	210/206/210
65+ *Free-living*	11	6	7	495/467/477
65+ *Living in an institution*	52	21	11	147/134/141
Female aged (years)				
1.5-4.5	9	n/a	17	476/-/463
4-6	8	24	9††	82/61/63
7-10	16	18	2	143/119/99
11-14	4	20	14	171/155/128
15-18	9	30	27	169/159/136
19-24	7	27	16	53/47/53
25-34	8	17	8	157/154/157
35-49	10	18	12	298/296/298
50-64	7	8	8	210/206/210
65+ *Free-living*	9	15	9	474/446/451
65+ *Living in an institution*	39	30	10	135/119/122

† percent less than 20µg/l; †† percent less than 15 µg/l

Thresholds

Haemoglobin (g/dl): 1½-6 years (male & female) <11.0
7 years + male <13.0
7 years + female <12.0

Iron saturation %: 4 years + (male & female) < 15

Serum ferritin (µg/l): 1½-4½ years (male & female) <10
7 years + male <20
7 years + female <15

Table 12   Mean vegetable, fruit and fruit juice consumption (grams per day) (NDNS)

Population group	Vegetables	Fruit	Fruit Juice	Total fruit, vegetables and fruit juice*	Number of subjects (unweighted)
	g/day	g/day	g/day	g/day	
Males & Females					
1.5-4.5 years	39	50	37	126	1675
Males aged (years):					
4-6	60	63	44	167	184
7-10	58	62	54	174	256
11-14	73	42	55	170	237
15-18	94	44	62	200	179
19-64	137	87	48	273	766
65+ Free-living	123	97	24	244	632
65+ Living in an institution	102	60	9	171	204
Females aged (years):					
4-6	58	65	49	172	171
7-10	69	68	53	190	226
11-14	70	48	53	171	238
15-18	101	54	61	216	210
19-64	132	103	47	282	958
65+ Free-living	109	96	25	230	643
65+ Living in an institution	83	61	19	163	208

* Not calculated using 5-a-day definition. May include more than one portion of fruit juice and more than one portion of beans/pulses

Table 13   Average consumption of oily fish* per week (NDNS)

Gender and age	Mean (g)*	Number of portions**	Number of subjects (unweighted)
Males and females aged 1.5-4.5 years	5	<0.1	1675
Males aged (years)			
4-6	6	<0.1	184
7-10	5	<0.1	256
11-14	10	<0.1	237
15-18	10	<0.1	179
19-64	51	0.4	766
65+ Free-living	85	0.6	632
65+ Living in an institution	29	0.2	204
Females aged (years)			
4-6	7	<0.1	171
7-10	8	<0.1	226
11-14	5	<0.1	238
15-18	7	<0.1	208
19-64	50	0.4	958
65+ Free-living	47	0.3	643
65+ Living in an institution	28	0.2	208

*Excludes canned tuna. Includes recipe dishes
**One portion is about 140g

Table 14   Mean consumption of oily fish* per week by females aged 11-49 years in LIDNS

Age (years)	Mean (g)*	Number of portions**	Number of subjects (unweighted)
11-18	7	<0.1	215
19-34	21	0.2	483
35-49	63	0.5	494

* Excludes canned tuna. Includes recipe dishes
** One portion = 140 grams

Table 15   The percentage of women classified by BMI as overweight and obese in the NDNS

Age (years)	Overweight or obese	Obese
15-18	–	–
19-24	39	14
25-34	44	16
35-49	54	23

Table 16   The percentage of women classified by BMI as overweight and obese in LIDNS

Age (years)	Overweight or obese	Obese
11-18	34	19
19-34	47	23
35-49	60	34